Social Relations and
Chronic Pain

Plenum Series in Rehabilitation and Health

SERIES EDITORS

Michael Feuerstein
Uniformed Services University of the Health Sciences (USUHS)
Bethesda, Maryland
and
Anthony J. Goreczny
Chatham College
Pittsburgh, Pennsylvania

ENABLING ENVIRONMENTS: Measuring the Impact of Environment on
Disability and Rehabilitation
Edited by Edward Steinfeld and Gary Scott Danford

HANDBOOK OF HEALTH AND REHABILITATION PSYCHOLOGY
Edited by Anthony J. Goreczny

INTERACTIVE STAFF TRAINING: Rehabilitation Teams that Work
Patrick W. Corrigan and Stanley G. McCracken

SOCIAL RELATIONS AND CHRONIC PAIN
Ranjan Roy

SOURCEBOOK OF OCCUPATIONAL REHABILITATION
Edited by Phyllis M. King

A Continuation Order Plan is available for this series. A continuation order will bring delivery of each new volume immediately upon publication. Volumes are billed only upon actual shipment. For further information please contact the publisher.

Social Relations and Chronic Pain

Ranjan Roy
University of Manitoba
Winnipeg, Manitoba, Canada

Kluwer Academic/Plenum Publishers
New York, Boston, Dordrecht, London, Moscow

Library of Congress Cataloging-in-Publication Data

Roy, R. (Ranjan)
   Social relations and chronic pain/Ranjan Roy.
      p.   cm. — (Plenum series in rehabilitation and health)
   Includes bibliographical references and index.
   ISBN 0-306-46496-9
   1. Chronic pain—Social aspects. I. Title. II. Series.

RB127 .R677 2000
616'.0472'019—dc21

                                                      00-046621

ISBN: 0-306-46496-9

©2001 Kluwer Academic / Plenum Publishers, New York
233 Spring Street, New York, N.Y. 10013

http://www.wkap.nl

10 9 8 7 6 5 4 3 2 1

A C.I.P. record for this book is available from the Library of Congress

Printed in the United States of America

To Margaret

PREFACE

This book is an extension of my 1992 book entitled *The Social Context of Chronic Pain Sufferers.* Many ideas nominally explored there are elaborated in this volume, which is an attempt to fill a major gap in the chronic pain literature. Although there has been a virtual flood of new works on the medical and psychological aspects of chronic pain, such enthusiasm is somewhat muted in relation to the social environment of the patient. Although there is universal recognition among pain experts that biological, psychological, and social factors influence the experience of pain, the social component (for reasons that are unclear) has failed to attract much attention.

The need for a book focused on social relations is obvious. The patient is not merely a carrier of symptoms. There is a large social reality in the background of each patient; that reality can have multidimensional consequences, from the way pain is perceived to serious financial hardship and other sources of stress, complicating treatment, management, and, ultimately, the prognosis. Clinicians recognize the value of incorporating the social dimension in the overall evaluation and treatment of the patient. This book attempts to accomplish that task.

In order to achieve that objective, this volume addresses many important elements in the patient's social environment—the most significant being the family. Beyond the family, for a vast majority of patients, work represents a major source of economic security and self-esteem. Job loss, common in this population and a major cause of much personal and family distress, needs critical examination. Similarly, much of a patient's energy involves dealing with formal organizations, such as workers' compensation board, insurance companies, etc. Many patients describe their experiences with these organizations as humiliating and degrading, thus adding to their already compromised sense of self. Interaction with the medical world is perhaps the most important activity for the patient; disappointment with health professionals is pervasive since many patients do not find significant relief from their pain. Worse still, there is much doubt about the cause of the pain. This book purports to bring to the fore issues and problems that profoundly affect the sense of well-being of our patients, and what actions are necessary to ameliorate or minimize their sense of powerlessness.

The book is divided into chapters, as follows.

Chapter 1: Nature of Social Dislocation for Chronic Pain Sufferers

This chapter addresses the vast changes commonly experienced by chronic pain patients, including loss of employment, loss of income, marital tension, family dysfunction, social isolation, and persistent pain. An ecological framework lends itself to a proper examination of the changes in the patient's social environment, and the foregoing problems are explored through case illustrations and relevant literature where available.

Chapter 2: Cost of Chronic Pain

In addition to the social environment, the economic consequences of chronic pain—for example, low-back pain—are astronomical. The relevant literature is reviewed to acquaint the reader with the cost of chronic pain and its social and financial repercussions.

Chapter 3: Myth and Reality of Family Function

Family relations of chronic pain patients are often troublesome. Over the past two decades, a respectable body of research and clinical literature has evolved. While there is significant evidence of family dysfunction in this population, it is not universal. Many families in the face of great odds continue to function well. This chapter explores both aspects.

Chapter 4: Impact of Parental Illness and Pain on Children

Are the children of chronic pain patients more vulnerable to psychological distress, depression, and other health and psychosocial problems? The empirical evidence is critically reviewed. In addition, case vignettes are presented to show the trials and tribulations that children encounter as a result of parental illness. A common problem that many children report is the distancing from both the sick parent and the well parent for different reasons.

Chapter 5: What Happens to Spouses?

This chapter focuses exclusively on marital relations with a focus on the repercussions of having a chronically ill partner. Evidence exists of a higher rate of depression and other psychosomatic problems in the spouses of these patients. Clinical evidence shows that the spouses of chronically sick patients are confronted with many more responsibilities, less support, and demoralization. These issues are examined by means of a thorough review of the literature supplemented by case illustrations.

Chapter 6: Family Intervention

This chapter presents an overview of family intervention literature followed by an account of an actual family therapy involving a chronic pain patient.

Chapter 7: The Nature of Social Support

Social support has emerged as a critical element in maintaining an individual's personal and social equilibrium. There is much research evidence to show the protective function of social support against morbidity. Recovery from illness is hastened through social support. This chapter reviews the benefits accruing from social support in general and its relevance to chronic pain. Its clinical significance in the well-being of the patients is highlighted.

Chapter 8: Chronic Pain Patient and the Occupational Role

Sadly, job loss is a common experience for chronic pain patients. Homemakers' functions are seriously compromised. By reviewing the concepts of illness behavior and sick role, we discuss the social, psychological, and deeply personal concerns generated by loss of occupational role. In addition, the outcome of chronic pain treatment literature is reviewed to determine how often return to work is used as a measure of treatment success. A case is made that for many patients such a measure is unduly hard, and a variety of measures is required to assess successful outcome correctly.

Chapter 9: Dilemma of Injured Patients: What Entitles Them to Compensation?

This chapter reviews the adversarial relationship that often exists between patients and the formal services primarily designed to ameliorate or minimize the negative consequences of chronic pain and job loss. Secondary gain emerges as a major issue. The validity of this concept is judged by reviewing the relevant research literature with special reference to chronic pain patients. A great deal of misunderstanding stems from a poor conceptualization and understanding of the chronic pain syndrome, which is often equated with malingering. This view becomes a major source of distress for many patients. Strategies for dealing with this issue are discussed.

Chapter 10: The Patient and the Medical World: Mrs. Kramer's Journey through the Medical System

The relationship of the patient to the medical world is complex. At the very heart of this complexity is the uncertain nature of the diagnosis of the pain complaint. A patient's veracity about the severity and persistence of the pain symptom is often challenged. It is not uncommon for patients to be given a psychiatric label, which most resent. When patients arrive at the pain clinic, they have virtually exhausted the medical specialties and are often very angry with the medical profession. The pain clinic represents their last hope since conventional medicine, by and large, has failed them. These problems and others are discussed through the eyes of one patient.

I received a great deal of help from many friends in bringing this project to conclusion. I would like to express my special thanks to my friends Robert Chernomas, Brian Minty, Ramesh Tiwari, and Harvy Frankel, without whose advice and guidance my job would have been considerably harder. My friends and colleagues at my pain clinic provide me with ongoing intellectual sustenance for which I remain indebted to them. I owe a very special thanks to my old friend Gunther Semelka, past director of our pain clinic, for his unfailing belief in me. I received a grant from the University of Manitoba Faculty of Social Work Endowment Fund for which I am deeply grateful. My wife, Margaret, as usual, acted as my in-house editor and adviser, and she has my deepest love and gratitude. Of course, without the cooperation and active participation of many patients, this book could not have been written. I cannot thank them enough.

CONTENTS

Contents

LIST OF TABLES AND FIGURES

TABLES

FIGURES

Chapter 1

NATURE OF SOCIAL DISLOCATION FOR CHRONIC PAIN SUFFERERS

INTRODUCTION

Many conflicts emerge in the lives of chronic pain sufferers. Most of these conflicts are unanticipated, and almost all contribute to the patient's misery. This chapter shows that coping with pain is only one of the many problems which collectively have profoundly negative consequences for the patient. Changes for the worse generally experienced by a chronic pain patient are legion. This chapter tells the story of a patient who found herself in conflict with almost all the organizations that were basically there for her benefit. Her story unfortunately is all too common and will sound very familiar to clinicians working with this population.

THE CASE OF MRS. ABRAMS

The case of Mrs. Abrams, age 43, not atypical in a pain clinic setting, is discussed to show the sheer impact of chronic pain on every aspect of her being. As her problems are identified, they will be assessed against the published literature.

Mrs. Abrams' developmental history was unremarkable. She came from a middle class background, was a good student, and eventually trained as a public health nurse. She married and had two children in quick succession. However, her marriage was a disaster. Her husband was physically abusive, and eventually she left him. She remarried, again to an abusive man, but quickly extricated herself from this relationship.

She entered a new relationship, and life seemed to be reasonably stable until she had an automobile accident. This accident was the beginning of her descent into chronic patienthood and long-lasting conflict with every system whose primary function was to help people like Mrs. Abrams.

Mrs. Abrams and the Medical World

Mrs. Abrams's journey through the medical world, first in search of a diagnosis and then a cure, was representative of what many of our patients report. Before this major accident, she was involved in another automobile accident, in which she sustained a whiplash injury from which she made complete recovery. She also had a long history of migraine, which was well controlled with medication.

Her second accident left her with restricted neck movement. One of her physicians noted that she had developed degenerative osteoarthritis of the cervical spine, which would cause periodic pain and disability and time off work. She chose to return to work for financial reasons, but was unable to continue. She had numerous psychological investigations, the conclusion of which was that she was too invested in her medical condition, and steps were required to help her disengage from pain behaviors. A cognitive-behavioral-oriented rehabilitation program was recommended by medical and psychological personnel engaged by her employer's insurance company. The disagreement between these medical opinions was at the root of Mrs. Abrams's legal problems with the insurance company. Despite clear organic finding, the pain was seen as out of proportion with the existing pathology. The psychological explanation that she was too focused on her pain, etc., left her feeling rejected and not believed, and, in rare instances she was even accused of malingering.

We now briefly examine the reasons for this state of affairs. A more detailed survey is given in Chapter 10. It is noteworthy that at one point Mrs. Abrams's was diagnosed with fibromyalgia.

At the heart of this problem is the mismatch between the patient's complaint of intolerable pain, on the one hand, and the lack of, or insufficient, physical evidence to account for the pain, on the other. The patient is sent from specialist to specialist, getting the same message that the results of the medical investigations were either negative or, at best, inconclusive. What might account for this state of affairs? It is perfectly reasonable to assume that the early investigations are legitimate, but at some point physicians begin to question the veracity of the pain complaint. Research into physicians' attitudes in this area yield complex results. For example, one body of research confirms that agreement between physicians and patients on treatment yields a better outcome (Cook and Roy, 1995). In relation to the chronic pain patient, problems commence at an earlier stage, namely dispute over the diagnosis. That might explain a common observation that by the time a patient is seen at a pain clinic, his or her attitude to the health care profession is somewhat soured.

On the other hand, many patients are reluctant to accept psychological and psychosocial attribution (Eisenthal *et al.*, 1994). This problem is more complex than appears at first glance. To begin, a patient presents with complaints of unremitting pain. Pain is a signal for underlying disease, hence the patient's unswerving belief that there must be a physical reason for this pain. Frequently this journey, in the Canadian health care system, begins with the family physician, who as a starting point might refer the patient to an orthopedic surgeon, as was the case with Mrs. Abrams. His findings that she had osteoarthritis seemed unrelated to the accident, but he was concerned about Mrs. Abrams's headaches and sent her to a neurologist. The patient went through another set of investigations only to be told that she had nothing to worry about. By this time the patient is more convinced than ever that the root cause of her pain was caused by the accident. In the meantime, her emotional state was becoming unstable. Psychiatric consultation was recommended but rejected out of hand. She had seen a psychiatrist during her abusive marriage and had scanty respect for that profession.

Evidence exists that when a physician adopts a psychotherapeutic attitude characterized by empathy and appreciates the psychological reasons for resistance, the patient is more likely to follow the physician's recommendation (Berg, 1987). However, Potts and associates (1986) found that a lessening of a patient's concerns was more strongly associated with favorable outcomes. That, unfortunately, is not a common experience among chronic pain patients. Generally, having exhausted all medical options, the patient is referred to a pain clinic by a specialist or by the family physician.

Belief in somatic rather than psychological cause for pain is commonly observed in this population. This either/or perspective rooted in Descartian duality of body and mind combined with built-in fear and prejudice about mental illness creates an optimal condition for hostility between chronic pain patients and their physicians. Besides, the patient's sense of credulity is seriously challenged at the mere suggestion that such suffering could be a product of the mind. This is not an easy concept to grasp even among health care professionals, let alone our patients. "How could that be? I am not imagining this pain. It is real. Do you think I am crazy?" Every clinician in a pain clinic setting has heard these questions. Patients then generally feel accused of lying about their pain. These and related issues are explored in Chapter 10.

Violon (1982) observed that "during the interminable journey through the medical mill, the pain is still present, severe or torturing. Moreover, the patient feels lost, more anxious, or frankly desperate. The more anxious or depressed he becomes, the more violently he feels that pain. Progressively, he loses his status as an independent human being and becomes an object of care, sent from one practitioner to another, being palpated, pricked, radiographed, submitted to a variety of technical examinations, to innocuous or painful diagnostic means, and varied therapeutics, but less often carefully listened to and understood" (Violon, 1982, pp. 32–33). This judgment of the medical profession may be viewed as rather harsh, yet from the patient's point of view Violon's observation is almost generous.

To return to Mrs. Abrams, at some point, in addition to her osteoarthritis in her cervical spine, she was diagnosed with fibromyalgia, a diagnosis that is still surrounded by a certain amount of controversy and cynicism. Her contact with the medical profession was otherwise filled with disappointment and despair. Although there was acknowledgment that the accident had caused some measurable level of distress, the injury was not seen as sufficiently damaging to prevent her from working. There was disagreement on this issue between the pain clinic physicians and the medical and psychological personnel working for the insurance company.

Naming a poetential cause—might even minimally account for the pain—is not only desirable but imperative. To be simply told, as is often the case, that there is "nothing wrong" is anathema to the patient, due to unremitting pain, inability to function on a daily basis, and a mounting sense of doom. The truth is that much is wrong. The reasons may not be clear, but a denial that much is wrong only adds insult to injury.

The World of Work

Mrs. Abrams continued to work following her accident, but then as a result of deteriorating health and increased demands at work, she took medical leave. She returned for a short while on a part-time basis, and finally resigned her position. This loss was highly significant to our patient.

Loss of employment for many patients represents more than loss of livelihood, which in itself is not a trivial matter. The costs of underemployment and unemployment are substantial and are discussed in Chapter 2. The social cost of unemployment is also considerable. Health problems, suicide, substance abuse, abusive behavior, family conflicts, and even marital breakdown have all been associated with unemployment. We briefly describe role theory (elaborated in Chapter 8) to appreciate this loss.

The basic tenet of role theory is that all of us have prescribed and ascribed roles. Through performing these roles, we develop some sense of who and what we are. Evolvement of the sense of identity is the heart of this theory. Worker, parent, student, child, etc., are definitions of ourselves, embedded in which is our obligation and duty. The loss of any of these identities involves—indeed demands—a redefinition of the individual. When Mrs. Abrams resigned her position, she lost what we all consider to be a vital element of her sense of self. She lost her place in society as a valued member of a helping profession. Above all, she lost a simple, yet a core, component of her identity. Redefinition of the self was called for, but the answer was far from acceptable. The answer in her case was that of a chronic patient. This radical change in identity extracts an enormous psychological cost. Some patients may experience relief, but not Mrs. Abrams, who took exceptional pride in her profession. She felt humiliated, unfairly treated by the world, sad, and even grief-struck and very angry. Her emotional state was in great turmoil. Her loss of self-confidence was telling.

Intellectually, she was able to appreciate the hardship and pain she experienced in performing her duties. Her family physician and the pain clinic staff were supportive of her inability to do her job. Yet, all this support was meaningless to her when she finally decided to quit her job. The emotional cost of this decision was enormous. For a very long time she could not bring herself to talk about this matter without breaking down and crying. For Mrs. Abrams, this was more than a job loss. It represented some kind of personal defeat in which society had conspired against her. How else can one explain a minor whiplash injury culminating in a major psychosocial and medical disaster.

In this context a brief allusion to the concept of "reference group" may be worthwhile because it helps explain a particular kind of emotion expressed by Mrs. Abrams. Simply put, the concept confirms our desire for indispensability. As parents of young children, as supervisors of graduate students, as health care professionals we not only have the need to be needed, but we may feel indispensable. This job loss left Mrs. Abrams with the feeling of being un-needed and unwanted. These feelings are tied to the universal desire to be indispensable, which gives us purpose and the drive necessary to function on a daily basis. For a health care professional, this indispensability in a very real sense is connected with patient care. Patients need us and cannot do without us. On our part, we do our utmost to provide that care. This feeling adds to our individual and collective sense of indispensability. Intellectually, we may all be aware of our dispensability, but psychologically the need for the reference group that enhances our sense of indispensability in our lives is essential. Mrs. Abrams described her job loss in melodramatic metaphors. She was saying, essentially, that if she could not work the purpose of her life was over.

Chronic sick role is a derivative of sick role originally conceptualized by Talcott Parsons (1951). Sick role in its original form stipulated a matrix of obligations and duties. A sick person could expect to receive care, nurturing, and treatment, but he or she is obligated to get well and resume normal activities within a certain period of time. With chronic illness this obligation becomes hugely complex. A patient's functional capacity is often unclear, but the general consensus is that given the limits of physical and or mental disability, a patient could still function in some areas, though not in others. However, this whole process is far from smooth, and can be complicated by the patient's personality, the behavior of the patient's intimates, and society's expectation. There is also the risk of a gap between the health care professional's assessment and the patient's own, which can add to feelings of mutual hostility. Gallagher and Wrobel (1982) noted that, compared to an acute sick role, there is increased autonomy and responsibility for maintenance of health within the chronic sick role. The role occupant's responsibility is to maintain the highest possible level of health and functioning. Furthermore, since the chronically sick patient's activities occur outside the sphere of intensive acute medical care, that person's life will embrace values and functions other than sheer compliance with medical goals and procedures.

What was Mrs. Abrams' functional capacity? Could she work or couldn't she? Was the degree of disability she was claiming justifiable on the basis of her injury associated with the accident? This was more than a medical issue. It became the focus of legal wrangling and much recrimination. It is noteworthy that at this early stage of her disability, she was vacillating between normal and chronic sick role. There was acknowledgment that she had osteoarthritis of the cervical spine. The debate was twofold: (1) Was it caused by the accident? (2) Could it justify her claim of disability? It seemed that she was likely to lose on both counts.

Mrs. Abrams and the World of Insurance

Mrs. Abrams experienced some of these conflicts. Her automobile accident set her on a journey that was far from predictable. It brought her into conflict with the Kafkaesque world of insurance. The basis of this conflict was whether the accident was the cause of her subsequent health problems. The Canadian province in which she resides has a state-operated automobile insurance corporation which is the sole insurer for automobiles in the province. In general terms, the insurance scheme runs well and serves the citizenship of the province with efficiency and speed. That unfortunately was not the case with Mrs. Abrams.

The insurance company (IC) refused to accept any liability for her health problems, simply stating that her chronic pain condition(s) was unrelated to the accident. Cognitive dissonance is often the outcome for patients when they receive this type of message from insurance companies or worker's compensation boards (WCB). There was, for example, no doubt in Mrs. Abrams' mind that the accident was the beginning of her serious health problem. She was a well-functioning human being up to that point. The fact that the accident completely changed her life is an incontrovertible truth. If the accident and ensuing pain did not cause her present state, what did?

Thus began a three-year journey. The IC demanded that she go through a rehabilitation program and, perhaps, retrain for a job. This was a concession of IC in the sense that, while still rejecting any direct connection between the accident and her ill health, they were prepared to help her to be rehabilitated.

She barely survived the rehabilitation program, which she found demeaning mainly because "they" failed to recognize her as a highly intelligent woman of some accomplishment. She left the program feeling thoroughly humiliated, with her morale at an all time low. Thus started a prolonged legal battle. It took several years before the IC and Mrs. Abrams came to a financial settlement, a condition of which was that she absolved the IC of any further liability. It is also noteworthy that the IC was adamant in its assertion that there was no scientific evidence to link trauma-related accident and the emergence of fibromyalgia or osteoarthritis.

In a recent newspaper article on Gulf War Syndrome, chronic fatigue syndrome, multiple chemical sensitivity, and fibromyalgia were described as lacking an objective explanation, which leads "many doctors to reject a patient's disability as spurious or dismiss symptoms as psychological" (*Guardian Weekly*, January 3, 1999). Dismissal of psychological symptoms with such readiness is indeed telling. At the heart of many conflicts between our patients and WCB and insurance companies is the unwillingness of these organizations to accept psychological distress and, sometimes, psychiatric disorder as resulting from work-related or other accidents.

It is not an exaggeration to state that much of the dispute between chronic pain patients and their insurance companies, workers compensation boards, and other financial institutions is analogous to Mrs. Abrams' case. In the absence of clear-cut evidence that the accident caused or contributed to the worsening of a particular disease, secondary gains or malingering are invoked to deny claims, and psychological distress related to trauma is often minimized. It ought to be recognized that the literature on chronic pain and malingering has established that malingering is extraordinarily rare in this population.

Secondary gain is a complex concept, which unfortunately has assumed a rather simplistic interpretation, namely, individuals exaggerate symptoms to avoid work and claim disability benefits or some other kind of financial gain. The truth is that a vast majority of patients' loss of income is barely compensated by these benefits. Hence, they stand to gain nothing financially because the benefits fall far short of their income. Secondary gain is a psychological phenomenon. One example of secondary gain is when pain extricates a patient from unsatisfactory sexual relations with the partner. The level of pain may not explain this behavior. The patient rarely, if ever, is aware of this behavior. If it is a conscious act, it is no longer in the category of secondary gain. Much misunderstanding surrounds these concepts, and often contributes to an adversarial relationship between patients and financial institutions and even health care professionals. Several studies have shown that settlement of financial claims does not end the patient's pain and suffering. If money was the sole motivation for faking or exaggerating pain, then logic dictates that following the financial settlement the symptoms will become redundant, but that is not the case (Tunks, 1990). It was certainly not so with Mrs. Abrams, who has not yet been able to return to her profession and continues to attend the pain clinic for ongoing management of her pain. Her psychological state is somewhat improved, and she is no longer in desperate financial straits, but her life remains much diminished. These issues are explored in depth in Chapters 8 and 9.

Mrs. Abrams and the Family

A significant body of literature on the family functioning of chronic pain sufferers has evolved over the past 20 or more years. The general consensus of that research is that chronic pain has profound negative impact on many aspects of family functioning, ranging from communication, role performance, intimacy, ability to show positive emotions, and so forth (Thomas and Roy, 1999).

To say that chronic illness in a family member is capable of profoundly changing how that family functions is merely stating the obvious. The extent of these changes depend on the degree of disability, role of the family member, life stage of the family, etc. If a mother with young children is disabled through a chronic illness, the adjustment needed for this family to function satisfactorily is considerable. On the other hand, in a family, such as Mrs. Abrams', with grown daughters and a supportive partner, adaptation to their new reality may be less challenging. The point, however, is that adjustments in family functioning are inherent whenever a prevailing homeostasis is disrupted by a chronic disorder in one of its members.

These changes are often adaptive, and many families make the necessary adjustment to maintain family functions. The chronic pain and family literature provides evidence that supports this perspective (Basolo-Kunzer *et al.*, 1991; Nicassio and Radojevic, 1993). Yet many families experience an inordinate amount of adjustment problems and in effect become somewhat dysfunctional in many areas. Two aspects that tend to fall victim to chronic pain are communication and role function. Communication suffers as family members protect the patient and over time lose the ability to express their negative emotions; the patient also develops the feeling of increased dependency and loses her or his right to express all feelings (Roy, 1989). This creates an environment where much remains unsaid and gives rise to much tension. As far as role function is concerned, when a patient falls victim to a chronic disorder such as that of Mrs. Abrams she is not only made unemployable, but is unable to carry out some daily chores. The patient not only has more time at hand but is increasingly able to do less and less, which often creates family dissension. Others are required to assume the roles and responsibilities discarded by the patient. They may refuse or do so unwillingly and resentfully. Again, these factors further contribute to the unhealthy state of the family. Many aspects of family functioning are discussed in Chapters 3–5.

The family is generally viewed as the major source of support for any of its members in need. This truth is certainly not universal since many families are dysfunctional or filled with dissension. In addition, the spouse may engage in pain-reinforcing behaviors, which is detrimental to the patient. This problem is discussed in Chapter 7. However, the importances of a supportive family and its benefits are well illustrated in the literature. McFarlane *et al.* (1983) showed that in the face of negative events the only significant factor in preventing morbidity was a caring spouse. These marriages were characterized by reciprocity and mutual caring and respect.

Obviously, when a family member is sick or disabled, family functions are often compromised. A sick child may take parental attention away from other children, or illness in the mother may significantly jeopardize the well-being of the whole family. Over the past 25 years, we have learned much about the family functioning of chronic pain sufferers, and will discuss it presently. But a great deal of evidence exists to show that many families are adversely affected by a chronic pain sufferer.

Mrs. Abrams's entire life was completely altered in less than a year from her accident. She changed from a very competent woman in virtually every aspect of her life to a chronically sick one who seemed to be in conflict with everyone and everything. Such massive disruptions in her life could not leave her family situation unaffected. One of the most significant changes was from being the main breadwinner in the family to having virtually no income. While she fought the IC, she refused to be on social assistance. Her husband had his own health problem and worked only sporadically. This family was on the verge of a financial catastrophe.

Through all this, Mrs. Abrams's husband remained her confidant and best friend. He was completely on her side and encouraged her to fight on. This level of spousal support has come under scrutiny in the literature, and is interpreted as undesirable because it promotes pain behaviors in the patient (Thomas and Roy, 1999). She acknowledged in retrospect that she could not have survived without the unconditional support from her husband.

Role changes introduced by chronic illness are contingent on level of disability combined with the value a patient might place on certain roles. We have observed that Mrs. Abrams lost one of the most cherished roles, that of a nurse. On the domestic front, her roles were somewhat less affected. The fact that her children were grown helped. The situation was further mollified by the attitude of her husband, who remained very supportive throughout her ordeal, and that he was home a great deal. He was happy to take over chores that Mrs. Abrams had found hard, such as vacuuming—a critical aspect of effective family functioning. Relieving the patient of chores helps to preserve essential family functions. The literature suggests that this area of family functioning comes under severe strain.

For Mrs. Abrams, however, a fiercely independent woman, who had left an abusive husband, had a profession, and raised two children almost single-handedly, changes in her family roles, however minor, were far from acceptable. Although objectively most of the family functions were maintained, she was deeply saddened, because even the slightest sign of disability filled her with forebodings of terrible things to come. Depression, demoralization, apprehension about the future, and preoccupation with the pain contribute to create considerable distancing between partners and between parent and children.

We now briefly speak about chronic pain and depression. The nature of this topic has changed over time. Over twenty years ago the discussion centered on whether idiopathic chronic pain was another manifestation of a mood disorder (clinical depression). Pain symptoms were ubiquitous in the clinical depression population and often masked underlying depression. The argument that chronic pain was a manifestation of depression was simply an extension of the prevailing wisdom that pain and depression coexisted; sometimes depression was the primary symptom and sometimes pain was. Because many chronic pain patients have common symptoms associated with depression such as anhedonia, loss of libido, sleep disturbance, etc., gives further credence to this argument.

Understanding the chronic pain syndrome has improved significantly. It is now universally acknowledged as a complex multifaceted syndrome with an intricate mix of biological, psychological, neurological, and social factors. Symptoms of depression remain common in this population. However, there are now three explanations for this situation: (1) Some portion of chronic pain patients do indeed suffer from clinical depression and chronic pain, both of independent origin (comorbidity); (2) many chronic pain patients develop dysthymia, or reactive depression in the old taxonomy, in response to the losses they incur as a consequence of their pain condition (e.g., Mrs. Abrams); (3) many chronic pain and medically ill patients have common symptoms of depression which could be misinterpreted as symptoms of a primary depressive disease.

In the bedroom, there was very little change because they rarely engaged in coitus, mainly bcause of Mr. Abrams' pathological obesity. Disruption of sexual activity is common, and sexual problems are legion in this population. Numerous studies attest to the fact that sexual function is a common casualty of chronic pain. The most common reasons offered are pain and depression. An added factor is enhanced tension between family members. In addition, complex dynamics often enter marital relationships and prevent partners from intimate behaviors. Couples lose their capacity for sharing their intimate feelings, and sex tends to recede far into the background. In therapy many couples express their great sense of loss of intimacy.

Depression and demoralization are not uncommon in the spouses of chronic pain sufferers, and they contribute to lessening or eliminating sexual activities. In many families if the husband and father is the patient, the upheaval caused by his disability is nothing short of disastrous. Much of the responsibility for keeping the family together falls on the wife with very little support from her partner. Indeed, there could be resentment over this transfer of responsibility. On occasion husbands will set out to sabotage or undermine the newly acquired authority of the spouse. Even without that kind of destructive behavior, many women feel very stretched and thoroughly demoralized. Loss of income is also a major contributor to the mounting tension.

Mrs. Abrams continued to carry out, not entirely to her satisfaction, many of her domestic duties. She learned not to overextend herself and, thus, avoided the cycle of doing too much followed by more pain and then being forced to give up and be demoralized. Objectively, given the magnitude of her losses, her family life remained more or less intact. However, it would be overly simple to ignore the financial hardship experienced by this family, which caused a fair amount of dissension between the couple. Mr. Abrams's inability to earn a decent wage was the main cause of this conflict. Besides, from Mrs. Abrams's point of view nothing was intact. Her assumptive world was destroyed by an event which at first sight was trivial (Fig. 1.1).

SUMMARY

The story of Mrs. Abrams is not atypical of many chronic pain sufferers who wind their way into a pain clinic setting. Her journey through various systems is summarized in Fig. 1.1. A relatively minor injury sets the course for chronic pain and despair. Other than the problem of pain, which itself is serious, many factors contribute toward making this journey even more painful and extraordinarily frustrating. Society is in some measure responsible for this state of affairs.

Modern medicine, with its total reliance on technology for diagnosis, takes a dim view of conditions that cannot be explained on solid scientific or objective clinical observations. If the condition is such that objective data may be insufficient or simply lacking, questions are raised about its very existence. Many of our patients face this problem with some degree of regularity.

Faced with the uncertain nature of the problem, psychiatric and psychological explanations are sought. This tends to lessen the legitimacy of psychological and psychiatric problems. Patients regard denial of a physical cause for their pain as demeaning and invocation of psychological explanation as rejection, or at least minimization, of their pain and suffering, or at worst simply questioning their veracity. Health care professionals require a language to address this issue. Lack of objective finding is not to deny existence of a problem. Rather, an explanation that acknowledges the suffering of the patient and the limits of medical science to explain the pain may be a more auspicious beginning. Psychological and psychiatric explanations are legitimate and need careful explanation, because to any pain patient such explanation appears farfetched. Linking psychological distress with pain does not agree with common sense. Most patients fail to appreciate such a connection.

It is a matter of some curiosity that institutions that exist to deal with loss of income, unemployment due to illness, or other kinds of calamities become a

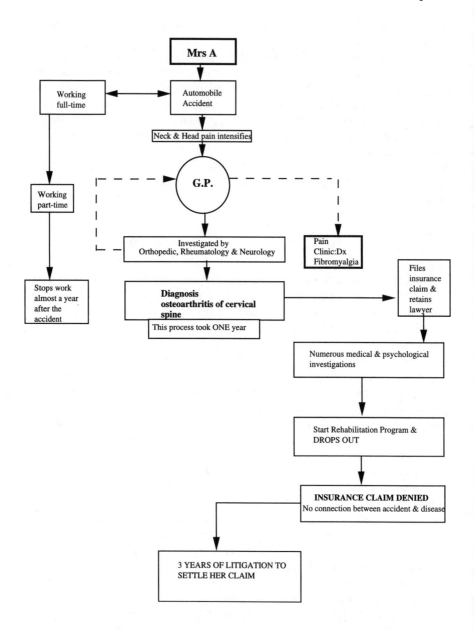

Figure 1.1. Mrs. A's journey through various systems.

major source of suffering for so many patients. There is no simple solution to this problem. On the other hand, if these institutions recognized, based on empirical evidence, that fakery and secondary gain, etc., rarely motivate people to seek financial gain, they will adopt an attitude that reflects understanding. On balance most patients lose a great deal more than they gain from some financial settlement. Mrs. Abrams, for example, has now permanently joined the ranks of the poor from a very middle class existence.

Notwithstanding, they have an obligation to investigate the matter, and again this can be accomplished without creating an adversarial relationship with its clients. Institutional culture often contributes to these undesirable attitudes. These attitudes require revisit and modification, which is happening in many Canadian centers, but yet not enough. Reviewing Mrs. Abrams's case, one has to wonder why it took so long to arrive at a settlement, and one is left with the lingering feeling that fairness of her claim was secondary to the institutional culture of distrust and creating maximum obstacles to any swift settlement, lest clients come to the wrong conclusion that the insurance company was soft or could be taken in.

The most drastic consequence for Mrs. Abrams's family was their descent into poverty. Lack of money was at the root of many of their problems. There were drastic changes in Mrs. Abrams's role, from a health care professional to a chronic patient. This had ramifications for her husband and daughters. But given the life-stage of her family, her grown daughters, and her satisfactory marriage, the actual family disruption from her illness was not overwhelming. In any event, the centrality of the family as a source of both stress and support demands that family issues of our patients should be kept in the forefront. However, as we shall see, the impact of chronic pain can be nothing short of devastating.

Chapter 2

COST OF CHRONIC PAIN

INTRODUCTION

Even to a casual reader, the social and economic costs of Mrs. Abrams's chronic pain condition must make an impression. The total cost of her medical investigation, her loss of employment, the fact that society lost a highly trained health care professional, financial ruin of the family, financial dependence of the family on the state, the emotional cost on the patient and her family were extremely high. In this chapter we explore two aspects of the cost of chronic pain. In analyzing cost, our focus will be on chronic low-back pain (CLBP) and the cost of another common consequence of chronic pain, which is unemployment. Mrs. Abrams's cost of medical investigations, including the cost incurred by her insurance company up to her referral to the pain clinic, was relatively modest. Her job loss and joining the ranks of "disabled" was quite telling.

Linton (1998) observed that "the socioeconomic impact (of chronic back pain) for the individual is often neglected.... The problem then is very prevalent and has great direct and indirect impact on society, the health care system, and above all the individual and her/his family." Of course the emphasis in the literature has been on the cost of medical intervention and days lost due to back pain. Linton (1990), in his review, cast a wider net to argue that the impact of chronic pain is much more than the preoccupation with the cost of medical care.

Numbers and statistics tend to mask great individual suffering and tragedy. In this chapter, while dealing with research studies, we shall not lose sight of our individual patients. The effects of Mrs. Abrams's pain, unemployment, financial difficulties, and depression are indeed related. The genesis of the problems can be traced to her intractable pain problem, and all the other issues tend to minimally complicate the clinical picture and demand that, for a comprehensive understanding of her circumstances, we carefully examine the social cost of chronic pain in a broader context then just monetary terms. To that end, we propose to explore the financial cost, but we also examine the cost of unemployment and its relationship to marital and family relation and depression. Depression is a particularly complex issue because our patients have many reasons to be depressed and demoralized. Chronic pain itself is capable of engendering or at least eliciting depressive symptoms.

When unemployment and financial and familial difficulties are considered, we begin to develop a more realistic appreciation of our patients' vicissitudes. In the first part of the chapter, we briefly review the financial cost of chronic low-back pain (CLBP), which is ubiquitous in Western society and serves as a reasonable prototype for chronic pain syndrome. In addition, CLBP patients are probably the single largest diagnostic group in most pain clinics. The main focus of this chapter is unemployment-related issues and how they tend to complicate immeasurably the clinical picture of our patients. We plan to address some of the socioeconomic factors related to unemployment and additional health consequences that seem to emanate from unemployment. It must be acknowledged that the literature on these topics on chronic pain population is very sparse, but through extrapolation we hope to show that unemployment and underemployment are key factors, when combined with chronic pain and debilitating disorders, in contributing to much misery, and explaining the collapse of the patient's assumptive world. We discuss the worker role and the emphasis on returning to work in multidisciplinary pain treatment programs in Chapter 8.

MEDICAL COST OF CLBP

Our reason for the rather cursory treatment of CLBP is that this topic is much discussed, and there is general consensus that medical cost alone for CLBP is astronomical. However, the literature on cost is not always clear and, indeed, contributes to the confusion. The confusion can be traced to the question, "what constitutes the cost?" The answer to this question is far from self-evident. Several studies include loss of workdays as part of the cost. In fact, two elements, namely social cost and medical cost, are generally evident in a great many studies.

Waddell (1996) noted that, despite much improvement in our knowledge and expertise for spinal pathologies, there continues to be an exponential increase in disability resulting from nonspecific low-back pain. He attributes much of this disability to the specialist-oriented management of CLBP in the United States, which involves high-tech investigation resulting in high cost. In addition, several investigators have found that a relatively few CLBP patients account for a very high proportion of the medical cost. A much earlier study reported that, while CLBP was often described as of obscure origin, sociological factors, such as wage and wage compensation, occupational characteristics, and marital and familial status, often removed some of the obscurity (Volinn, 1986).

Sociological factors were also noted by Valat and associates (1997), who observed that occupational factors substantially impact the cost determination of low-back pain. Blue-collar workers, men involved in heavy labor or in jobs that require effort beyond their physical ability, workers with low job satisfaction or poor working conditions, new employees, and employees who receive unsatisfactory ratings by their superiors are more likely to develop chronicity. In a study of nurses, Mitchelmore (1996) found that psychological and social consequences of back injury at work were very serious and generally ignored. Lack of opportunities for redeployment and the generally unsympathetic attitude of the employers significantly contributed to the nurse's ability to remain in the profession.

The actual medical cost of treatment for low-back pain has been difficult to establish. One study investigated the cost of each medical and surgical service received by low-back patients and a group with thoracic back pain, and provided at least a preliminary guideline for estimating the cost of investigation and treatment (Dreiser *et al.*, 1997). The actual medical cost of back pain in Germany was reported to be $8 billion per year, $2.2 billion of which was direct medical cost. Most of the cost was incurred in physician visits and diagnostic investigations (Bolten *et al.*, 1998). Only a fraction of the total cost was actually medical in nature. Again, the authors recommended intervention directed more at prevention, along with programs designed to return their patients to work rapidly.

Webster and Snook (1990) investigated 98,999 computerized records of insurance claims for low-back pain and estimated that medical costs represented 31% of the total costs; the total compensable cost for all low-back pain in the United States was estimated to be $11.1 billion. Large variations were found in cost between states. In a subsequent study these authors reported similar findings in terms of high cost of back pain and noted that most of the cost was related to indemnity (payment for lost time), 65.8% of the total cost. Their recommendation was that the primary goal of low-back pain management should be prevention or reduction of prolonged disability (Webster and Snook 1994). The cost of back pain in The Netherlands was estimated at 1.7% of the GNP. Of that cost 93% was indirect costs for absenteeism and disability (van Tudler *et al.*, 1995). In an earlier review of low-back pain management, Frank (1993) concurred that the "strategies to manage low-back pain must be long-term and preventive; and the responsibility to keep fit, maintain an exercise program, and remain relaxed so as to avoid physically straining the spine is that of the individual, not of the professionals." This view obviously disregards jobs that are inherently bad for the back.

The finding of excessive medical cost confined to a few patients was confirmed in a Swiss study (Jeanneret *et al.*, 1998). They found that 5% of low-back pain patients consumed 80% of the cost. Their suggestion for cost reduction was to improve diagnostic procedures and make careful selections for surgical intervention. Similarly, Frymoyer and Cats-Baril (1991) observed that the cost of back pain was $50–100 billion in the United States, and 75% or more of that figure was accounted for by 5% of low-back pain sufferers. Their contention was that these patients, who for the most part developed short-term or long-term disability, had problems rooted in psychosocial factors rather than disease determinants.

Additional information lends further credence to these findings. In an investigation of workers compensation for back pain, Hashemi and colleagues (1997) found that only 10% of low-back pain claimants were responsible for 86% of the total cost. Similar observations were made at primary care settings where a minority of low-back patients accounted for most of the cost (Engel *et al.*, 1996). They found that 21% of the total sample of 1059 subjects presenting with back pain accounted for 67.7% of the total cost. Persistent pain, disk disorder, and chronic pain grade were strong independent predictors of high total and high back pain costs. To prevent such costs, Engel *et al.* suggested behavioral interventions to target problems of persistent pain, depression, and general dysfunction. Such early intervention may prevent high utilization of health care resources. We review the outcome of treatment for chronic pain in Chapters 8 and 9.

Volinn and associates (1991) reported that not only does a small minority of low-back patients represent a huge portion of the cost, but some ineffective practices, such as surgery, have increased over the last 15 years in the United States. In fact, these authors go further in asserting that few treatments for low-back pain have proven to be more effective than a placebo. During the same period pain clinics have been busily advocating a more conservative approach to back-pain management.

Similar observations were made by Johnnaon and associates (1994). They cite several studies in support of their argument that much of the treatment for back pain was unnecessary or even detrimental. Borenstein (1995) also expressed concern about the overuse of surgical procedures in the United States, compared with 11 other countries. Besides, a great deal of the cost associated with low-back pain was not medical, but disability and delay in returning to work. He urged careful selection of patients for specific types of back surgery. Another factor contributing to high medical cost was identified by Liu and Byrne (1995). They found that overall utilization of health care services was higher for patients who were referred to subspecialists, and the cost of visits to them was also higher. Many patients not meeting MRI criteria were nonetheless accorded that test. Overall, 6% of the subjects who failed to meet either the criteria for referral to subspecialists or MRI accounted for 27% of the total charges.

Van Tudler and associates (1995) found similar trends in The Netherlands. They examined cost as direct and indirect. Direct cost included hospital care and costs, specialist care and costs, and primary care and costs. Indirect cost included cost of absenteeism and cost of disablement. Over half the expenditure of medical cost was due to hospital visits, suggesting extensive use of costly diagnostic procedures. Cost of hospital care due to back pain constituted the largest part of direct medical cost, estimated at $367.6 million. Musculoskeletal diseases were the fifth most expensive category for hospital care and the most expensive regarding work absenteeism and disablement. The indirect cost constituted 93% of the total cost of back pain. As an antidote to high medical cost and the belief that much low-back pain requires education and prevention, Frost and associates (1998) demonstrated the benefit of a fitness program and proposed a more active approach to treating chronic low-back pain. The benefits of a community-based nurse-delivered psychoeducation program was also demonstrated with a group of chronic pain patients (39% with CLBP) in a randomized controlled trial study (Le Fort *et al.*, 1998). The findings presented a picture of reliable short-term improvement. In those who were enrolled in the psychoeducational programs compared to a group of wait-list controls, the highest level of improvement reported was in physical role functioning. Overall improvement was 9% to 47%.

Summary

In this brief review of the literature several facts stand out.

1. The actual medical cost of chronic back pain is only a fraction of the social cost. This appears to be so in many countries.
2. There is a consensus that medical cost represents many unnecessary medical interventions which, for the most part, do nothing or little to alleviate pain but, in all probability, contribute to the iatrogenic factor.
3. Medical intervention must accompany social and psychological therapies because these factors seem to play a role in the genesis of back pain.
4. Prevention and back education should be the focus as far as low-back pain is concerned.
5. The high social cost is almost entirely attributable to short- and long-term disabilities associated with back pain.
6. Only a fraction of all back-pain patients account for a disproportionate amount of the medical and social costs.
7. Despite considerable advancement in the management and treatment of chronic low-back pain in modern pain clinics, its overall impact in reducing cost appears to be nominal. A major inference is that, despite these advances, physicians show a marked preference for conventional medical and surgical interventions many of which have been shown to be of little or no use.
8. Sociological factors inform us that this population is not particularly well educated, and, for want of a better term, belongs to the working class. That, by definition, puts them at a disadvantage in terms of their power and re-sources.
9. This extremely lopsided picture of a very few chronic low-back patients making a huge demand on insurance companies and workers' compensation

boards may, in part, account for much distrust and hostility between patients and these agencies. This latter issue is explored in Chapter 9.

COST OF UNEMPLOYMENT

The foregoing discussion leaves no room for doubting the very heavy financial cost of disability associated with chronic low-back pain. That unemployment is not a rare occurrence is familiar to all who interact with pain clinic patients. In this section we propose to go beyond the statistics and, first, present two case vignettes which depict great personal loss and humiliation in one, and family tragedy and suicide in the other; second, we examine the literature to develop an appreciation of one of the consequences of unemployment, namely depression. The reason for our focus on depression is simply that many chronic pain patients suffer from some level of depression or minimally present depressive symptoms. Unemployment may very well contribute to further aggravation of an existing condition or induce depression. Either way, unemployment adds another level of complication to the clinical picture of these patients, which we, as clinicians, need to take into account. We return to some aspects of this topic in Chapter 8.

Mr. Bloom, age 42, emigrated to Canada from a Mediterranean country and was successful in his chosen country. He was married with two sons and a daughter. His pain problems commenced with a work-related accident that injured his right hip and leg. Initially, this was no more than a passing inconvenience, but, as with so many chronic pain patients, his pain was not relieved but became more severe and led to associated disability. In six months he was totally incapacitated by the pain. Mr. Bloom then became extraordinarily angry with the medical profession, workers' compensation board, and, unfortunately, with his children. He became a family tyrant. The source of his anger was twofold: (1) persistent pain and loss of the breadwinner role, which held enormous importance for him. His inability to provide for his family drove him to distraction. Devastated by these changes, Mr. Bloom committed suicide two years after the accident.

The second case involved Mrs. Chambers, a 54-year-old woman, who presented with low-back pain of unknown origin. She qualified as one of those few CLBP patients who made extraordinary demands on medical and other resources. After an investigation that lasted almost a year, during which time she stopped working as a shop assistant, she was referred to a pain clinic, where she was diagnosed with fibromyalgia. She continues to be a patient at that clinic, and, despite the passage of several years, she mourns the loss of her job and remains psychologically quite distressed. To Mrs. Chambers, unemployment meant almost total social isolation and loneliness. Her workplace was the very center of her social life.

These two cases show very different responses to job loss. More importantly, they give us an insight into the social and financial complications that are inextricably tied up with job loss, which make coping with pain that much more difficult.

Unemployment and Chronic Pain

A major Canadian study (D'Arcy and Siddique, 1985), involving 14,313 subjects drawn from a Canada Health Survey's national probability sample of 31,688 people, revealed the far-reaching consequences of unemployment. Significant health differences emerged between the employed and unemployed: the unemployed showed a higher level of distress, great short- and long-term disabilities, numerous health problems, were patients more often, and used proportionately more health services. Interaction effects of socioeconomic status and demographic variables showed an association of employment status and emotional health. The blue-collar unemployed were more prone to physical illness in contrast to white-collar workers, who seemed more vulnerable to emotional distress. Low-income unemployed who were the principal wage earners were the most psychologically distressed. It is noteworthy that a pain clinic population is well represented by this last group. It serves as a double-edged sword because insufficient education has been noted to be one of the barriers to returning to work among individuals suffering from arthritis and musculoskeletal disorders (Straaton et al., 1996). Fear of layoff and unemployment has also been associated with low-back strain injuries, resulting in lost time. Non-low-back injury rates were highest during periods of high turnover and no layoffs (Clemmer and Mohr, 1991).

That the unemployment rate is high among back pain patients was recently reported in a comparative study of headache and back pain patients which was designed to grade the severity of chronic pain for use in community samples and study of primary care patients (Stang et al., 1998). The sample consisted of 662 headache and 1024 back pain subjects. Over the study period of three years, 13% of headache subjects and 18% of back pain subjects were unable to obtain or keep full-time work due to their pain condition. Among the employable, 12% of headache subjects and 12% of back pain subjects were unemployed. Grading of chronic pain emerged as a significant factor in predicting disability, and the highest grade of chronic pain predictably showed high levels of affective distress. Unemployment was strongly associated with pain grade. A major conclusion was that the likelihood of reduced labor force participation among primary care patients with headache was considerable and concentrated among the one out of five patients with poor long-term outcome. In addition, confirming an earlier observation, younger women and or poorly educated persons were the most vulnerable for unemployment.

A direct relationship among chronic pain, depression, and unemployment remains essentially uncharted territory. From a methodological perspective, depression as a result of unemployment would be hard to separate as simply depression; at least, depressive symptoms are common accompaniments of chronic pain. In fact, recent research has pointed out the complexities associated with diagnosing depression in patients with physical diseases using the most common depression inventory, the Beck Depression Inventory (BDI). The items for physical symptoms in the BDI might be confusing when determining depression (Soederman and Lisspers, 1997). The nonphysical components seems to be the best indicator of depression. However, Averill *et al.*, (1996), in an investigation of 300 chronic pain patients, found that among several factors, such as education level, marital status, and interaction between age and gender and depression, unemployment was associated with increased depressive symptomatology. They concluded that employment was an important role and its loss could produce serious psychological consequences. Work status, among other factors, accounted for significant variance in depression scores. This finding is important because it confirms the day-to-day observations of clinicians who regularly encounter patients devastated by job loss.

Von Korff and associates (1992), in an investigation of grading severity of chronic pain, found that "for each pain site, chronic pain grade measured at baseline showed a highly statistically significant and monotonically increasing relationship with unemployment rate among other factors." In other words, pain severity predicted unemployment, functional limitations, depression, poor self-rated health, and overuse of opiates and health care services. A higher unemployment rate was also reported in a community-based Swedish study which examined all first referrals to a pain clinic over a two-year period. Referrals presented common sociodemographic characteristics, a higher rate of unemployment as well as higher representation of immigrants; in addition, the high rate areas for referral compared to the "average" showed a higher percentage of people in need of social security. In short, a disproportionate percentage of the chronic pain population was poor, unemployed and of foreign extraction (Ektor *et al.*, 1992).

Emotional distress caused by psychosocial factors as a result of unemployment was also reported in a controlled study of 83 chronic pain subjects and 88 healthy controls (Jackson *et al.*, 1998a). After controlling for length of current unemployment and number of pain sites, several psychosocial measures, such as structured and purposeful time use, perceived financial security, and social support from formal sources, were the most powerful predictors of emotional distress. Structured and purposeful time use emerged as the most significant predictor of emotional distress for both groups. This study goes substantially beyond just considering the direct effects of unemployment; it addresses in a comprehensive way some of the consequences of unemployment and their power to predict emotional distress. The double jeopardy of chronic pain and unemployment is a major source of concern for patients and clinicians (Fig. 2.1).

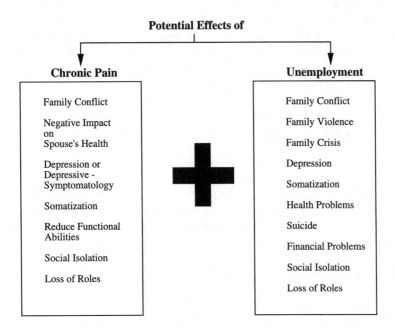

Figure 2.1. Double jeopardy of chronic pain and unemployment.

Unemployment and Depression

The social costs of unemployment, even by conservative estimates, are very high. They range from family discord to suicide to child and spousal abuse. Poor health is a well-known outcome of unemployment. The Canada Health Survey (D'Arcy and Siddique, 1985), in a most comprehensive study of its kind, conclusively demonstrated the far-reaching consequences of unemployment on health, which were confirmed by a major American study (Linn *et al.*, 1985). In a prospective study of 300 men assessed every six months, men who became unemployed were compared with those who remained employed. After unemployment, somatization, depression, and anxiety were significantly greater among unemployed men.

In the preceding section, in addition to discussing the cost of chronic pain, we alluded to the high unemployment rate among the pain clinic population and CLBP patients. Study after study confirms that the social cost, which includes unemployment and disability for this population, is high. The rationale for separately examining the impact of unemployment in this population is that a problem (pain) that starts out as a medical concern can soon become a major social issue, and the nature of the original medical problem is made far more complex by a patient's social realities. If unemployment is indeed capable of producing depression, then the chronic pain population is faced with double jeopardy in the sense that depression, or at least depressive symptoms, has been long associated with chronic pain, and unemployment with its own noxious effects only enhances the risk of depression in this population. It should be recognized that the literature on unemployment and depression is huge, and we plan to present only a select review of it.

We referred to a study by Averill and associates (1996) in the previous section. This study is important because it is one of the few that investigated the impact of unemployment on depression. Three hundred patients were randomly selected from a sample of 1000 patients referred to a pain clinic for evaluation and treatment. Of the subjects, a remarkable 67.7% were unemployed. A statistically significant association was found between work-related variables and Beck Depression Inventory. This study was unequivocal in its finding of an association between unemployment and increased depressive symptomatology. Unemployment as a trigger for depressive symptoms received considerable support.

A Swedish study also reported a higher level of depression in a group of unemployed women compared to an employed group (Hall and Johnson, 1988). Their results showed that even when controlling for social support, stressful life events, and marital status, depression on the basis of the BDI was higher in the unemployed group. Age also appears to be a factor in engendering negative emotions as a result of unemployment. (Recall that middle-age people constitute the bulk of chronic pain patients.) Rife and First (1989), in a study of 73 unemployed workers age 50 and over, found pervasive feelings of social isolation, embarrassment, mild depression, and a generally low life satisfaction. In contrast, younger participants in the same sample who also had higher levels of education and longer periods of unemployment reported greater adjustment problems. It is well known that older persons not only have a harder time obtaining reemployment but are also more susceptible to layoffs. Shame appears to be an integral part of being unemployed, and generates guilt and poorer mental health, even clinical depression (Eales, 1988; Smith, 1985).

Since the chronic pain population tend to be among the long-term unemployed, a Norwegian study may have special relevance (Claussen *et al.*, 1993). In a group of 270 long-term unemployed Norwegians, the prevalence of depression, anxiety, and somatic illness was 4–20 times higher than a control group of employed people at baseline. A striking finding of this study was that chances of reemployment were reduced by 70% among those with a psychiatric diagnosis.

Unemployment affects not only a victim's mental health, but also the mental health of the spouse. Longitudinal data from 815 recently unemployed job seekers and their wives or partners revealed that financial strain caused by unemployment significantly affected the depressive symptoms in both partners (Vinokur *et al.*, 1996). This, in turn, caused withdrawal of social support, thus creating a vicious cycle of marital discord and depression. The impact of chronic pain on the partner is discussed in Chapter 4.

Unemployment and Suicide

In a major review of the literature on health and unemployment, the authors concluded that although poor health could lead to unemployment, the reverse is equally true (Dooley *et al.*, 1996). They found confirmation in aggregate-level studies on association between unemployment and suicide rates over time. At an individual level, surveys of laid-off workers showed increased psychiatric problems, such as depression and substance abuse. Unemployment was also found to be a predictor in a group of hospitalized parasuicides (Petrie and Brook, 1992). Overall, prediction of suicidal behavior was increased by including age, history of previous attempts, and unemployment.

Unemployment and suicide or suicidal ideation have been reported in India, Australia, and Ireland (Kelly *et al.*, 1998; Latha *et al.*,1994; Lyster and Youssef, 1995; Morrell *et al.*, 1993). In the Indian study of 58 individuals who attempted suicide and 60 normal controls, the significant factors that distinguished the two groups were their exposure to a number of life-events. Among the life-events, unemployment emerged as a significant contributor to suicidal attempts.

The Irish study revealed that single status, unemployment, and lower socio-economic status were the three most significant factors that accounted for suicidal attempts (Lyster and Youssef, 1995). An Australian study of prevalence and predictors of suicidal ideation and past suicide attempts in a sample of HIV-positive and HIV-negative subjects revealed that among factors associated with suicidal ideation were current psychiatric disorder, external locus of control, and current unemployment (Kelly *et al.*, 1998). Another Australian study that investigated the relationship between suicide and unemployment throughout the twentieth century showed that the highest rate of male suicide occurred during the Great Depression (Morrell *et al.*, 1993). In fact, the trend was for the male suicide to show sharp rises during all periods of high unemployment, while the number of female suicides remained more or less stable.

Plant Closure and Depression

An Italian study investigated the power of being laid off from work to engender depression (Rudas *et al.*, 1991). Laid-off workers as compared to a control group of full-time workers were found to be more susceptible to depressive symptoms.

Dew and colleagues (1992) reviewed the literature on the effects of unemployment among women, and conducted a prospective study to investigate the effects. They found that the duration of layoff was significantly related to depressive symptoms even after effects of pre-layoff psychological symptoms, social support, and occupational stress were considered. Results showed a pattern of interaction between unemployment and demographic factors, showing differential vulnerability to unemployment. However, a British study showed that no association was found between social class and scores on health measures in middle- and working-class men who had been unemployed for 18 to 24 months (McKenna and Payne, 1989). Unemployment led to both groups reporting equally poor perceived health. A point to be noted is that this study was on "perceived" health rather than actual health status.

In a large-scale study, workers from 4 GM plants which were being closed and 12 from plants remaining open were investigated for the psychological effects of being laid off, compared to those who remained employed (Hamilton *et al.*, 1990). Less-educated workers (it is noteworthy that blue-collar workers abound in the CLBP group in particular and as pain clinic patients in general) and African–Americans were especially affected. Follow-up data showed that their more distressed mental health could not be accounted for by previous stressors. This study and the previous two tend to confirm that unemployment by itself is sufficiently noxious to put unemployed persons at risk for depression, depressive symptoms, or poor mental health.

Finally, we report a European study which investigated associations between unemployment, financial situation, and mental well-being (MWB) in a group of 135 employees of a factory that had closed (Viinamaeki *et al.*, 1993). A poor financial situation was associated with impaired MWB. This poor financial situation was accentuated by poor social support. Subjects who were uncertain about their future had more difficulty in coping than did others. This last study is telling because it summarizes many of the common problems encountered by chronic pain patients, namely, job loss, loss or decline in social support, and, often, serious financial hardship.

SUMMARY

This chapter has attempted to relate critical areas that affect our patients. While *prima facie* the cost of CLBP or chronic pain in general may not have the appearance of any direct clinical relevance, the truth is that from the patients' point of view there are several issues directly emanating from the cost issue. One is that only a fraction of CLBP patients account for most of the medical and a huge proportion of the indirect cost. How does that fact influence the outlook of insurance companies and workers' compensation boards when they encounter these patients? It perhaps, in part, explains the heightened tension that often exists between our patients and these agencies. Second, there is much evidence of over-use of diagnostic services for CLBP, the net result of which may very well be a strengthening of somatic belief to which a vast majority of our patients subscribe. After much investigation many of these patients have a difficult time believing the objective negative findings and tend to view the medical profession as untrustworthy, uncaring, and even hostile. Minimally, they develop the unfor-tunate belief that the extent of their pain is minimized or that they are simply not believed.

Concerning the socioeconomic factors, the most significant are the low education and lower socioeconomic standing of many CLBP sufferers. This last issue is especially relevant in relation to options for reemployment. As a relatively weak segment of the population, they also confront powerful institutions, from the medical establishment to insurance companies. Their power of negotiation is, by definition, restricted, and their encounter with these powerful bodies only enhances their sense of powerlessness. There is no easy solution to this dilemma other than to recognize that the socioeconomic status of CLBP patients in many of our pain clinic patients is an added burden. The advocacy role of the pain clinic professionals to redress the power imbalance assumes great importance with these patients.

Chapter 3

MYTH AND REALITY OF FAMILY FUNCTION

INTRODUCTION

Is it inevitable that as a result of chronic pain a family's ability to function within "normal" bounds is compromised? Although the literature leaves little room to doubt the negative effects of chronic pain on the family, we shall visit this complex question from a fresh perspective. When a family member is chronically ill, what should be his or her optimal level of functioning? Can a patient with chronic pain be expected to function, for instance, in sexual relations without difficulty? If not, how do we determine what may be the satisfactory level of sexual activities? Almost all major studies point to family disruptions, including sexual dysfunction caused by chronic pain. Study after study reveals that the family functioning of chronic pain patients is seriously compromised.

What is far more challenging to determine is a reasonable level of functioning. Common sense indicates that families with chronic pain patients are less likely to function at the level of normal families. Yet chronic pain families are measured against these normal families, and as long as the chronic health problem persists it is reasonable to assume that family functioning will not resemble the "norm." For example, a person whose leg is amputated below the knee will probably learn to walk but not to run. It is grossly unfair—even silly—to compare such a person's mobility with that of a healthy individual. Hence, to compare a family with a chronically sick member to normal families is at the very least problematic. Such comparison fails to consider that the chronic sick role is more than likely to produce major changes within a family system and requires a different level of adaptation to accommodate the needs and deficits of the patient.

The conventional approach fails to make any accommodation for the sick member, and research repeatedly informs us about the departure of these families from the norm. We shall review that literature with a different question in mind: We know that chronic pain families show marked deficiencies in many areas of family functioning, but can we address the question of what their "adaptive" level of family functioning should be? Perhaps the family cannot run, but can its members learn to walk? More importantly, how do health care professionals recognize that they are walking?

We review the recent literature on family functioning of chronic pain patients examined from a systemic (interactional family functioning) point of view and we illustrate the problems of using a tool such as the McMaster Model of Family Functioning (MMFF) to assess family functioning with chronic pain.

LITERATURE REVIEW

Bebbington and Delemos (1996) made an interesting observation which is relevant to this discussion. They noted that, despite all variety of marital problems for chronic pain patients reported in the literature, "marriages of chronic pain patients are more stable (longer lasting) than average." They speculated that this finding could be understood in terms of systems theory.

Findings of systems-oriented investigations into the family functions of chronic pain sufferers are less consistent in their negative findings than family investigations designed to investigate the impact of chronic pain on, for example, family members such as spouses and children. Our review of recent literature considers studies that support high prevalence of family dysfunction as well as those whose findings are to the contrary. Relevant issues are examined to illuminate the mixed findings.

Kopp and associates (1995) investigated family functioning in a group of mothers with chronic headaches and CLBP. Mothers with chronic headaches were compared with pain-free mothers. In general, mothers with headaches as well as CLBP were reported as deficient in many aspects of family functioning compared to normal controls. On the other hand, a closer scrutiny of the family functioning data based on the Family Environment Scale (FES) revealed a more complex picture. On the FES no significant differences emerged on 6 subscales out of 10 between the clinical and healthy subjects. As is frequently the case, the investigators were almost exclusively focused on those dimensions of family functioning where the differences were significant. That families were functioning within the "normal" range in most areas was not given any space. However, despite pain no significant differences were found in the following dimensions: cohesion, conflict, independence, achievement orientation, intellectual orientation, and control. Significant differences were found in expressiveness, active–recreational orientation, and moral–religious orientation. Could it then be claimed, based on these findings, that, despite pain, these families remained functional in most aspects of family life?

One positive finding is worthy of further attention. The CLBP and headache families were significantly less active in their free time than was the control group. Not only is this finding predictable, but it is almost inevitable that chronic pain will interfere with activity level. A more pertinent question is that, given their disability, what should be an acceptable level of free-time activity? Another issue is how does chronic pain in the mother compromise the overall activity level of the family? These questions were not addressed by Kopp *et al.*

Another study on the family functioning of chronic pain sufferers also utilized the FES but with very different findings than Kopp *et al.* (Naidoo and Pillay, 1994). Fifteen women with CLBP were compared with 15 healthy controls for family functioning. Significant differences were found on the following subscales of the FES: cohesion, conflict, independence, and organization. This contrasts with Kopp's investigation, which found significant differences in expressiveness, active–recreational orientation, moral–religious emphasis, and control.

There is no simple way to reconcile the differences because both studies included CLBP subjects. One significant difference was that many subjects in the Naidor–Pillay study were living in extended families, which would affect overall family functioning. This was a South African study, and while the ethnic background of the subjects was not revealed, cultural factors may be relevant in accounting for the differences. Nevertheless, the central observation is that these 15 CLBP families were, in the main, indistinguishable on 6 of the 10 subscales of the FES. These two studies together show that family dysfunction for the same diagnostic group and gender, on the basis of the same assessment tool, cannot be predicted with any degree of certainty. Second, and this point is often not adequately addressed, families appear to remain functional in most aspects of family functioning.

Romano and his colleagues (1997) used the FES to compare family functioning of 50 chronic pain patients and 33 control subjects. This was a complex study, and only the data relevant to this discussion is presented. Only 5 of the 10 subscales of the FES were used "in order to decrease the assessment burden on couples and because the study focused on relationship and family system issues." Of the 5 subscales (cohesion, expressiveness, conflict, organization and control), the pain patients reported significantly lower cohesion and higher control scores compared to the control group. Lower cohesion was suggestive of a patient's reduced ability to help and support; higher control indicated the need for rules and procedures to deal with demands of illness. On the other hand, expressiveness, which denotes a family member's ability to express a range of emotions, conflict, which might indicate anger, aggression, and tense situations among family members, and organization, which reflects the importance of clear organization and the importance of family activities and responsibilities, were not significantly different for the pain patients than for the control group.

One can argue that, given the overlapping nature of the subscales, effective functioning in, say, organization may seem, *prima facie*, irreconcilable with a compromised level of functioning on cohesion. Or does it simply suggest that family functioning does not lend itself to neat categorization, and a certain amount of overlap is inevitable? If the question is, How well do the pain families function compared to the controls? The answer is, at the very least, equivocal. Another notable point was that the areas of dysfunction were at variance with the Kopp *et al.* studies and Naidoo–Pillay studies. In short, there was no consensus about the aspects of family life that may be at risk due to chronic pain.

We now report one of our own studies involving 52 chronic pain patients and their spouses whose couple functioning was assessed with the Family Adaptability and Cohesion Evaluation Scale (FACES III Couple Version) (Roy and Thomas, 1989). We reported significant agreement between the couples in terms of marital dissatisfaction, but found them wanting in virtually every aspect of couple functioning. A closer scrutiny of the data somewhat alters that perspective. We noted that family adaptability, family cohesion, and family stability were compromised in various degrees.

We revisit the same data with a somewhat altered perspective. The combined score of the couple in Family Adaptability was 30.9, placing them just within the chaotic range (from 29 to 50), and just missing the flexible range from 25 to 28. Similarly, with Family Cohesion the combined score for the couples was 41.35, placing them in the desirable "connected" category. Finally, the couples were in the midrange category in Family Stability. In keeping with our hypothesis, these couples were found wanting, and we concluded that "the patients as well as their spouses provided powerful evidence of marital discord." A review of the data might demand softening of that stark conclusion. In Family Adaptability, couples were barely in the abnormal range; the Family Cohesion score placed them in the most desirable category; and Family Stability was in the midrange (not the most desirable nor the least). Couple functioning was not ideal, but was it, as we had concluded, mainly dysfunctional?

We now examine in some depth two studies that failed to show any family dysfunction in chronic pain families (Basolo-Kunzer *et al.*, 1991; Nicassio and Radojvic, 1993). Basolo-Kunzer and associates compared family functioning in a group of 117 headache patients and their spouses with a control group of 108 married couples without pain. They tested several hypotheses, two of which are relevant here. First, there would be differences in family cohesion, protectiveness, adaptability, and satisfaction between chronic headache couples and couples without chronic pain. Second, there would be differences in marital adjustment, satisfaction, conflict resolution, and sexual relationships between the headache couples and couples without chronic pain. FACES III was used to measure family cohesion, protectiveness, and adaptability. The Dyadic Adjustment Scale (DAS) was used to measure marital adjustment.

The first hypothesis was rejected because no significant differences emerged between the clinical and control groups. This was an astonishing finding in view of pervasive opinion and research findings to the contrary. The range in scores for headache couples on the FACES III was 21–93 (M=64.8, SD=9.9); for the control couples it was 42–97 (M=47.8, SD=9.0). In other words, scores for both groups resembled FACES III normative data. However, it ought to be recognized that 43 headache couples were not functioning in the normal range. Yet, extreme cohesion and extreme adaptability, suggestive of serious family dysfunction, was evident only in five headache couples. Similar data was not provided for the control group.

The second hypothesis failed to receive validation. The score for the headache couples on the DAS was 35–143 (M=111.6, SD=17.1), and for the control group was 52–141 (M=108.4, SD=16.8). These differences failed to attain statistical significance. A score below 100 on the DAS is indicative of marital distress. A total of 20% of the headache group and 24% of the control group scored below 100, thereby suggesting marital difficulties in both groups. Headache as a factor contributing to marital distress received only nominal support since more subjects in the control group reported marital difficulties.

Another study that failed to find any significant family dysfunction in clinical samples of chronic pain sufferers was reported by Nicassio and Radojevic (1993). The sample consisted of 44 rheumatoid arthritis patients and 46 fibromyalgia patients. Family functioning was assessed by the FES. No significant differences were found between the two clinical samples. Comparing these samples with the normative sample ($n=1125$) showed they were "highly comparable." In short, no significant differences emerged. In relation to family functioning the clinical samples, contrary to the expectation of the investigators, were functioning within the normal range. A later study by Nicassio and associates (1995) involving 122 fibromyalgia subjects confirmed their earlier finding that these patients functioned within the normal range of FES on the cohesion subscale, the only subscale used in this investigation. These studies are summarized in Table 3.1.

These last two studies raise a number of interesting issues. Can families sufficiently adapt to chronic illness to maintain normal family function? Although these two studies attest to that, even the investigators were surprised by the findings. The two studies involved different diagnostic groups, mainly white, mostly female, and relatively well educated. It is highly speculative to suggest that these factors influenced the outcome. However, the absence of family dysfunction in three diagnostic groups with chronic pain only adds confusion to the overall picture. The studies suggest that chronic pain and normal family functioning are not mutually exclusive.

This perspective is problematic, and goes to the heart of the central question in this chapter. Is the most effective or desirable form of family functioning for chronic pain families the same as "normal" families? The degree of disruption caused by chronic illness, adaptation to chronic sick role for the patient, reorganization of the family around the lost roles and responsibilities of the patient, financial resources, pre-morbid family functioning, and life stage of the family are

Table 3.1. Comparison of Family Functioning Between Clinical and Normal Groups

Investigator	Pain sites or diagnosis	Subjects	Controls	Instrument	Significant differences between clinical and control groups
Studies using FES					
Nicassio (1993)	RA & FM	44 & 46	Normative	FES: 10 subscales	No differences
Naidoo (1994)	CLBP	15	15	"	Cohesion, conflict, independence and organization
Kopp *et al.* (1995)	chronic headache & CLBP	12 / 12	12	" / " / "	expressiviness, active recreation, active religious, and organization
Romano *et al.* (1997)	chronic pain	50+50 spouses	33	FES: used 5 of the 10 subscales of FES	control and cohesion
Studies using FACES III					
Roy & Thomas (1989)	chronic pain	52+52 spouses	no controls; compared with normative scores	FACES III	mixed outcome
Basolo-Kunzer (1991)	chronic headache	117+117 spouses	108 married couples	FACES III	no differences

important areas of investigation in any clinical assessment of families with a chronically ill member. Different instruments for family assessment incorporate some or none of these elements. In other words, some areas of clinical import such as life-stage issues, financial security, and pre-morbid functioning are rarely incorporated. Besides, as shown by the following case illustration, clinical observations and judgments are often at variance from "effective" family functioning based on "objective" evaluation.

THE MMFF AND A CASE

The McMaster Model of Family Functioning (MMFF) was developed by Epstein *et al.* (1981) to assess normal family functioning. Using university students as their subjects, they identified several major areas of family functioning (Westley and Epstein, 1970). Each area is assessed on a continuum from effective to ineffective and is divided into two distinct categories: instrumental and affective. The goal of therapy is to enable the family to move from the ineffective range to the more effective. The question that this model does not seem to address is whether improvement in the direction of "effective" functioning is either possible or even desirable in all circumstances.

For example, an individual with chronic rheumatoid arthritis should not be compared with a healthy individual. Indeed it may be deleterious to health for that person to engage in certain activities, being quite incapable of carrying out some simple or routine chores. Hence, he or she needs to adapt to a level of functioning commensurate with the disability of rheumatoid arthritis. The McMaster Model fails to allow for this important phenomenon. In effect, a family harboring a chronically sick person must function at the same level as a healthy family for it to be described as effective.

A review of the research conducted by the McMaster group reveals a pattern of results which minimally raised important questions about the underlying assumption of what may constitute effective family functioning. Families of schizophrenics for example were found to be functioning within normal limits of effective family functioning, whereas families of unipolar depressives and alcoholics were in the abnormal range (Miller *et al.*, 1985). Many normal families gave evidence of ineffective functioning on some of the dimensions. Finally, one study with stroke patients found that the couple functioning returned to normal levels after a relatively short period following a cerebrovascular accident (Bishop *et al.*, 1986). In all studies, authors suggested caution in interpreting the findings due to methodological considerations. The central point is that the findings are mixed, and a tentative conclusion is that illness in a family member does produce lasting changes as far as family functioning is concerned. A contradictory conclusion is that families can indeed function in the effective range of the McMaster Model despite significant and major problems, such as schizophrenia or stroke.

The use of this model in research with a psychiatric population has been extensively reported. Some of the refinements in methodology have yielded complex results. A key finding in an investigation of maternal mental illness was that "variation in the conceptualization and measurement strategy for risk and family functioning affects the conclusion of research" (Dickstein *et al.*, 1998). Another study investigating family functioning with wide-ranging psychiatric disorders and healthy control concluded that, regardless of the diagnosis, acute mental illness in a family member was a risk factor for poor family functioning compared with control families (Friedman *et al.*, 1997). Two more studies involving depressed subjects reported that patients with "good family functioning at hospitalization generally maintained their healthy functioning and were likely to recover by 12 months the patients with poor family function" and second, patients with poor family functioning were likely to experience higher levels of depression and generally poor prognosis (Keitner *et al.*, 1995; Miller *et al.*, 1992).

Together these studies indicate movement in the right direction. Depression is not automatically equated with poor family functioning, and the relationship between psychiatric disorders and family functioning is bidirectional; that is, depression affects family functioning, but the reverse is also true. The most important result of the few studies cited here, and by many more that are not cited, is that family functioning is not an automatic victim of psychiatric disorders. In fact, the relationship is highly complex. This level of sophistication in methodology is not yet found in the chronic pain family research.

The efficacy of the MMFF to evaluate families of chronic pain has been reported by Roy (1988, 1989). The findings have been consistent in that almost all aspects of family functioning were found wanting. Through the process of studying families by using the McMaster model, a number of interesting issues have emerged, and serious questions have arisen about the desirability of "effective" family functioning as defined by the MMFF. It will be demonstrated here through a case example that what may be defined as effective within the model may not be the most desirable adaptation that families establish as their optimal levels of functioning and, most certainly, will be at variance with those of normal families. More significantly, for disabled families to emulate normal families may prove to be deleterious to their overall well-being.

We used the MMFF to assess the case of Mr. and Mrs. Donald (Epstein and Bishop, 1981). The MMFF identifies six areas of functioning: (1) problem solving, (2) communication, (3) roles, (4) affective responsiveness, (5) affective involvement, and (6) behavioral control. Functioning in each of these areas is assessed on a continuum of effective to ineffective. Space does not permit an elaborate discussion of the MMFF. Suffice it to say that we have used this model extensively and have reported on its strengths and weaknesses (Roy, 1989, 1990). To illustrate, we report on two critical dimensions of family functioning, namely, roles and communication, to simply show that on the basis of the assessment a family may appear ineffective, yet from a clinical perspective the family was actually coping well under a very stressful environment.

Mr. Donald, a retired senior civil servant, was suffering from chronic low-back pain and herpes zoster. He was considerably disabled by the latter. A conjoint session with Mr. and Mrs. Donald revealed a checkered marital history, considerably predating his current health problem. Mrs. Donald attributed their "poor" marriage to his poor health due to emphysema and clinical depression, afflictions he had suffered throughout his adult life. However, his poor health did not prevent his success in his profession, as he rose to a very senior position. They also had a 20-year-old daughter with Down's Syndrome, who lived at home.

Both parents harbored considerable guilt over the birth of their mentally challenged daughter, but Mrs. Donald expressed considerable feelings of recrimination. She received very little help from him in raising their daughter, and his involvement in family affairs was, at best, peripheral. The perception of Mr. Donald's poor health had a profound effect on his roles and responsibilities within the family. He remained an excellent provider. At the point of assessment at the pain clinic, their relationship resembled a caregiver–patient relationship. We now examine two aspects of their relationship, namely, roles and communication.

Roles according to MMFF: The model stipulates that effective functioning is a necessity for a family to fulfil all its duties and obligations. This model, like all other tools for family assessment, however, makes no allowance for persons who may be physically or intellectually compromised. Roles constitute a topic of some complexity in the context of chronically sick persons and their families. Problems usually are associated with the inability of the sick person to perform certain roles, which may range from occupational to many family-related roles, such as parental or spousal. Many of the roles may be restored through rehabilitation, others may remain impervious to treatment, and still others may even be contraindicated. Such losses can and do have profound effect on the family system, often creating tension, and certainly demanding realignment of roles.

Role functioning for the Donalds was very distorted. It may be instructive to consider some of the key aspects of role functioning to fully appreciate the extent of disruption, and the necessary adaptation that had to occur to maintain the family system.

Provision of Resources

This was not an area of concern for the Donalds, an upper-middle-class family who were able to maintain a comfortable lifestyle even after Mr. D.'s retirement. He had a substantial pension, owned their home, and had no debts.

Nurturance and Support: This involves the ability of the family to provide comfort, warmth, and support for family members. The nature of nurturance and support in this family was somewhat lopsided. Much of it was provided by Mrs. D. Her husband required a certain amount of reassurance and support, which Mrs. D. readily provided. He was very appreciative of the caring and nurturance he received, and he occasionally told her so. Both partners demonstrated a considerable level of caring for their retarded daughter, but the continuity was maintained by Mrs. Donald.

Adult Sexual Gratification

The McMaster model is very emphatic that a reasonable level of sexual activity is generally required, although Epstein and colleagues (1981) are cognizant that there may be situations where both partners may express satisfaction with little or no activity. The D.'s were very definitely in the latter category. Sexual activity never had a high priority in their relationship, and with the progressive deterioration of Mr. D.'s health it became nonexistent. Partners may express their satisfaction with little or no activity voluntarily or when it is imposed upon then by illness. These situations need to be distinguished.

Personal Development: This area of role functioning, according to the MMFF, is directly related to life stages. Many of the personal development issues concerned with healthy development of children and others are related to the career and social development of adults. The model is silent on the specifics of social development in adulthood as it proceeds or progresses through different life stages. It does not deal with how social development may be compromised and what may be the optimal level of development in the face of chronic illness in the family. The major task of the D. family was to adapt to the stress placed on the system by the presence of one chronically sick adult and an intellectually challenged daughter. Personal development issues for Mr. and Mrs. D. are somewhat moot. If acceptance is to be equated with growth, then both of these individuals showed considerable growth. Mrs. D. was able to adapt to her role of a nurse and a caretaker, and Mr. D. probably adapted a shade too well to the role of a chronically sick individual.

Maintenance and Management of the Family System

This area includes numerous functions such as leadership and decision making, boundary and membership functions with the outside world, behavior control functions such as disciplining of children, standards and rules for adult family members, management of household finance, and attending to the health needs of family members. This series of functions that purport to make a family a well-functioning system was almost solely the responsibility of Mrs. D. This was not by design but through necessity, since no one else in the family could fulfill these roles and obligations. Despite the seemingly unequal responsibilities, Mr. and Mrs. D. did not perceive this area as problematic. Their lives were governed by routine, and the family was at the stage where they were not confronted with major decisions daily. The only major decision that worried them considerably was the future of their daughter.

The other two critical areas of role functioning are role allocation and role accountability. Role allocation is concerned with assignment of tasks, and role accountability ensures that those tasks are fulfilled. These areas were not problematic for the D. family. Their daughter had some nominal chores which she carried out without too much difficulty. Most of the other tasks were carried out by Mrs. D.

Were the members of this family successful in role functioning? Mr. D. was certainly well adjusted to his chronic sick role, although he did wish to make some minor alterations. In the judgment of the pain clinic personnel, Mr. D. could function at a higher level. However, the essential role functioning tasks were carried out quite successfully, by Mrs. D. As far as could be ascertained, this family had no conflict in this area; the tasks were accomplished without much fuss, all three members knew what was expected of them, and Mrs. D. gave no evidence of resentment for her disproportionate amount of responsibility.

Note that on the basis of the McMaster Model or any of the main family assessment instruments, this family would have fallen short on several measures. Role functioning was lopsided. Mrs. D. carried an unfair share of the responsibility. Their intimacy was severely compromised, and the list of their family deficiencies was long. On the other hand, this family had adapted well. Without the willingness of Mrs. Donald to assume almost all major roles, it is more than likely that both her husband and the daughter would have been institutionalized. Far from ideal, clinically this family functioned well. The key point is that MMFF fails to recognize that, under certain conditions, "effective" family functioning is a far cry from the ideal.

It is noteworthy that in an investigation of environmental stressors in CLBP, Feurstein and associates (1985) found that families that scored high on the independence subscale of the Family Environment Scale

> "tend to be assertive and self-sufficient and to make decisions that do not involve other family members. Similarly, families high in organization tend to be dependent on family structure for planning activities and responsibilities. In such environment, pain patients may receive little support and attention, which necessitates pain behavior as a strategy to obtain such support."

"High" in organization is not a necessary condition for optimal family functioning. Situations may demand that "independence" be a desirable quality for effective family functioning. This perspective rooted in empirical evidence provides some support for our family to the extent that if Mrs. Donald had not assumed an independent approach to manage her family, the consequences could have been damaging to the well-being of the patient.

Communication

Communication is the exchange of information between family members, and the most effective form of communication is direct and clear. Assessing communication presented a special challenge from a clinical perspective so far as the D.'s were concerned. There was not a great deal of communication among family members. Much of what occurred was on mundane matters. They manifested an interesting complication that is often introduced into communication patterns among family members when one is chronically ill.

Mr. D. was reluctant to complain about his pains and discomfort because, as he put it, "it led to nowhere." He was concerned with not appearing to be overly demanding or complaining. Mrs. D. had her own problem with communication.

She responded to a question about her frustration, which she "must experience from time to time," by saying that, "If I open my mouth, it would be to complain. So I don't say anything." After a pause, she added: "I'm very used to the way we live. Nothing bothers me very much any more." When the therapist probed, asking, "How do you show your feelings to each other?" Mrs. D. replied that "we care about each other and that's really what matters." Communication to the extent it existed was perhaps clear and direct. Much remained unsaid. Both partners were protective of the other and themselves. They were afraid that openness could only cause conflict.

What should be the clinical considerations to judge the efficacy of communication between the D.'s? Do they function at the effective end of communication, or are they inept? How desirable is it for the D.'s to express all their thoughts and feelings openly and directly? Arguably, the pattern of communication was not ideal. On the other hand, there was clear recognition that complaining was likely to be unfruitful, and both parties recognized that fact and refrained from stating problems that could not be easily resolved. That could be seen as reasonable adaptation. From a therapeutic point of view, communication in this family seemed to be more than adequate. Their awareness of each other's feelings was the basis of avoiding certain topics, and could even be interpreted as a sign of caring. However, on the basis of MMFF, their communication could easily be described as ineffective on both counts of directness and clarity.

SUMMARY

Our brief incursion into the literature failed to shed much light on the basic question raised in this chapter. No two studies reported the same results. Some failed to find any differences between normal and chronic pain families. Differences in findings can probably be explained on methodological grounds and sampling issues. That, however, fails to resolve the central question: the assumption that the most desirable level of functioning for chronic pain families should be the same as normal families is simply absent in the research literature.

We also have not questioned that basic assumption, but have continued to confirm through our own research that, ideally, chronic pain families should aspire to resemble normal families. Yet, as clinicians we have found ourselves at increasing odds with the research findings. Two studies reported that the cohesion subscale of the FES was compromised for the pain patients. Perhaps, a brief examination of this finding may clarify the nature of the conflict between research findings and clinical goals. A chronic pain family's capacity to reorganize family life while making allowance for the patient is the real issue. This depends on several factors, a critical one being the loss of roles. If the patient happens to be the breadwinner and can no longer work, the level of adaptation required by this family is likely to be very demanding. Cohesion may never be quite the same, and in all likelihood adaptation in that respect may significantly differ from the cohesion subscale on the FES. Hence, we can argue that the desirable level of cohesion for chronic pain families will not be the same as normal families.

Through a case illustration we have attempted to show that family function is at the mercy of variables, such as the life stage of the family, degree of disability of the patient, unusual circumstances, such as having an intellectually challenged child, and pre-morbid issues. These issues mitigate against "effective" family functioning according to the MMFF. On the other hand, a careful analysis of the D. family reveals that adaptation of this family to an entire set of unpleasant realities, not to be found in normal families, required imagination, commitment, and, above all, a family organization that defied all definition of a well-functioning family. Yet this family was a well-functioning system, and much of the credit for that was due to Mrs. D.'s resiliency and Mr. D.'s accepting attitude.

It could be that we, as family therapists and researchers, have yet to learn a few lessons from the rehabilitation literature, which emphasizes the recognition of permanent physical deficits, which in turn determine the targets for improvement in the patient's functioning. We have yet to recognize the permanent damage to families caused by chronic pain, let alone the issue of acceptable level of recovery. As a consequence, we set unattainable goals and allow our intellectual muddle to expect chronic pain families to function like normal families. The task of researchers and clinicians is difficult. They must determine what constitutes effective family functioning in the face of chronic health problems. First, however, we must acknowledge that our present approach to ascertain effective family functioning for chronic pain families is flawed.

Chapter 4

IMPACT OF PARENTAL ILLNESS AND PAIN ON CHILDREN

INTRODUCTION

Rutter (1989) traced the pathways from childhood to adult life as influenced by varied childhood experiences and predictable childhood events in shaping the adult personality and behavior. Though childhood events and experiences have some long-term consequences, what those consequences might be continues to be a matter of speculation and research. The pioneering work of Freud and Bowlby recognized the centrality of childhood events and the certitude of their impact on the adult personality, yet recent research of Rutter and others has raised questions about such an inevitability. The vulnerability of children to various stressors in their environment has received considerable support in widely divergent fields, the death of a parent, separation and divorce, parental mental illness, and, to a lesser extent, parental physical illness.

In a pioneering study, Rutter (1966) compared the impact of parental physical and psychiatric disorders on the mental health of the children. His findings were complex, but much light was shed on the association between parental illness, especially of a chronic nature, and its propensity to inculcate psychiatric vulnerability in children. An unequivocal finding was that parents of children with psychiatric disorders manifested a significantly higher level of recurrent, as well as chronic illness, than parents with a physical illness. Chronic and recurrent parental physical illness was significantly higher among the children attending a psychiatric clinic than in matched groups of children attending dental and pediatric clinics. This ground-breaking study literally laid the foundation for systematically investigating the relationship between the health of parents and their offspring. Given the ubiquitousness of depression or depressive symptoms in chronic pain patients, we briefly review the parental depression literature, followed by parental disability and intractable chronic pain and their effects on children.

The parental role may be an important determinant of impact on the children. Does mother's illness produce more stress than the father's. While there is a mounting amount of research of maternal depression on children, literature on the father's impact is scarce (Jacob and Johnson, 1997). In their investigation of 50 depressed fathers, 41 depressed mothers, and 50 normal controls, the authors found that paternal and maternal depression were similarly associated with child adjustment problems and more impaired parent–child communication. In view of that fact, we briefly discuss the recent literature on maternal depression on children.

The evidence is far from conclusive. We shall demonstrate that many reports related to the children of chronic pain patients are methodologically wanting, and a close scrutiny of the data leads to a different conclusion from that reached by the investigators. In a major review of the consequences of parental illness on children, Roy (1990–1991) concluded that the two issues discussed in that review—incidence and prevalence of health problems in children of medically ill parents, and the risk factors for the children—could not be answered with any degree of certainty. Severity of the illness and the gender of the parent received partial validation as predictive of vulnerability.

Disability and depression are unfortunate accompaniments of chronic pain. This chapter explores the relationship among parental disability, parental depressive disorders, and parental chronic pain and their consequences on children's health. We do not engage in a truly critical review with focus on methodological issues. Our goal instead is to acquaint the reader with the current literature on these topics, this review is more a summary of our current state of knowledge. However, we do endeavor to make some judgment about the quality of research.

PARENTAL DEPRESSION

Depressive disorder is a relatively common psychiatric condition which is very amenable to treatment. Sadly, however, a portion of these patients tend to develop the chronic form of this disorder. This disease is more common in women than in men, and for that reason the literature on the impact of parental depression concentrates on mothers. This is evident in the following review, in three parts: (1) parental depression, (2) maternal depression and young children, and (3) maternal depression and older children.

Isaac and associates (1986) investigated 31 families with children who had stayed in foster care for a minimum of 12 months, and 26 families from the same district with children who had been under foster care for up to three months. Parents of children in foster care for the longer period were more likely to have received psychiatric treatment, and this correlated with a high rate of past and current psychiatric disorder in the total sample of parents. Parental psychiatric distress was an important factor in influencing children's admission and discharge from foster care.

Psychiatric effects of parental affective disorder on children has been reported by several authors. Beardslee *et al.* (1985) compared 37 children from 20 families with a history of affective disorder in one parent with parents of nine children from five families with no history of the disorder. A significantly high rate of general psychiatric impairment in the children of parents with major affective disorder and a marked amount of major depression according to the Diagnostic and Statistical Manual (DSM111) was found compared with the children of normal parents. Similarly, Keller *et al.* (1986) established that the more severe and more chronic the depression in parents, the poorer was the adaptive functioning and the higher was the level of psychopathology in their children.

Comparing the children of parents with unipolar and bipolar affective disorders, Kashani *et al.* (1985) found that children with unipolar parents were more vulnerable to separation anxiety and somatization and less likely to be alcohol dependent than were the children of bipolar parents. These results confirmed the high incidence of psychopathology among the children of parents with major affective disorders. Jary and Stewart (1985), in a somewhat unusual study, examined the records of 70 adopted and 70 nonadopted children for aggressive conduct disorder. Thirty-seven adoptees and 42 controls were diagnosed as having aggressive conduct disorder. They discovered that fathers of adopted children with aggressive conduct disorder were alcoholics and had antisocial personalities less often than the biological fathers of nonadopted children with the same condition.

Klein and Depue (1985) investigated 41 offspring of parents with bipolar disorder, between the ages of 15 and 20, and assessed their traits of obsessional personality. The cyclothymic offspring had significantly higher scores than the noncyclothymic offspring on the superego strength measure of obsessional traits. Obessionality was significantly correlated with affective symptom ratings which were not related to nonaffective behavior disturbance. The data indicated that obsessional traits may be associated with risks of bipolar disorder in the offspring of bipolar parents. Beardslee *et al.* (1985) had similar findings in nine children of parents with affective disorder.

A recent study of a 10-year-follow-up of 182 children from 6 to 23 years old of depressed versus non-depressed parents showed that the offspring of the depressed parents had higher rates of major depressive disorders and phobias (both at about three times higher), panic disorder, and alcohol dependence (about five fold higher) than children of non-depressed parents (Weissman *et al.*, 1997). The ages of 15–20 years were found to be the most vulnerable for offspring of both sexes. The authors concluded that parental depression increased the risk of depression in their children, that the course of the depression was protracted, and the children were vulnerable to a variety of psychiatric disorders.

This brief review reveals that children of depressed parents are vulnerable to childhood and later depression as well as wide-ranging psychopathology and behavioral and social disturbances. The reasons for the children's vulnerability are not always explained. It is conceivable that major mood disorders have a genetic basis, thus making the offspring susceptible. Beyond that, parental illness may create problems in child rearing. Parental bonding with the children may be loosened; the well parent's attention is also likely to be focused on the patient, further contributing to the child's feeling of isolation and rejection. These last two factors have considerable power to create emotional disturbances in children. A certain amount of parental neglect may be unavoidable.

Maternal Depression and Young Children

Several recent reports have appeared on maternal depression and its affects on young children. We present only a selected few. Interaction and attachment issues of mentally ill mothers with infants have received considerable attention. Weinberg and Tronick (1998) reported their preliminary findings for a group of 30 mothers in treatment for major depressive disorder, panic disorder, or obsessive–compulsive disorder. Their major finding was that maternal mental illness had a compromising effect on their interactions with their infants and on their infants' social and emotional functioning. Similar findings were noted in an earlier study, which also found that attachment insecurity of infants and preschoolers was significantly associated with maternal depression (Teti *et al.*, 1995). Furthermore, they reported, children without unitary, coherent attachment strategies tended to have more chronically impaired mothers than did children with coherent, organized attachment strategies.

Another study investigated the relationship between either unipolar or bipolar depression and personality disorders, and the relation of psychiatric problems to maternal caretaking behavior (DeMulder *et al.*, 1995). Mothers 23 to 45 years old with children, mean age 2.6 years at time 1, 5.5 at time 2, and 9.2 at time 3, were taken as subjects. The behavior of affectively ill mothers in interaction with their children was related to the mothers' personality disorder symptoms. This study concluded that personality disorder rather than depression alone accounted for the type of interaction mothers had with the children.

In the final study in this section, sleep problems were studied in 85 children and 75 of their older siblings whose mothers were diagnosed with unipolar or bipolar affective disorder or who had no current or past history of psychiatric illness (Stoleru *et al.*, 1997). Results indicated that sleep problems were more frequent and severe in children of affectively ill mothers. Younger children had more persistent sleep disturbance than their older siblings.

Maternal Depression and Older Children

This section is particularly relevant to our discussion because most of the children of pain clinic patients tend to be older. We briefly discuss some recent literature. Several studies reported on the impact of maternal depression on children from 7 to 27 years old (Hamilton *et al.*,1993: Tarullo *et al.*, 1994; Tisher *et al.*1, 1994). Tisher and associates compared 20 depressed children with 88 clinical nondepressed children and 55 normal children between 7 and 21 years old. Their findings were complex, but, for our purpose, a significant finding was that children and mothers in the depressed group reported more stressors than other children and other mothers, whereas fathers of children in the depressed group did not report more stressors. This study indicates that coping with depression is not necessarily a family affair where the burden is shared, but that the largest portion of responsibility in coping with depression falls on mothers.

Hamilton and associates (1993) examined communication styles of 64 children, 8 to 26 years old, of mothers with affective disorders and chronic medical illness, and 24 normal controls. A central finding was that the children's affective disturbance was linked to interpersonal deficits in affectively charged situations. The children's coping style was significantly influenced by the mothers' affective style rather than by the actual diagnosis of the child or the mother. In other words, the mothers' capacity for relating effectively with the children determined their coping. This phenomenon is commonly observed with pain clinic patients and their children. Many parents, despite their level of pain, remain connected with and concerned about their children, as opposed to others where the reverse is true. Generally speaking, family functioning at the pre-morbid stage is a major determinant of the parent (more specifically mother)—child relationship. However, functional problems in families are extraordinarily common and often complex when the mother suffers from depression and the father also has a history of psychiatric illness (Inoff-Germain *et al.*, 1997).

Another study that investigated communication between depressed mothers and their preadolescent and adolescent children reported that interactional difficulties were influenced by the maternal mood disorders as well as the child's problem status (Tarullo *et al.*, 1994). Another interesting finding was that mothers tended to be more critical and irritable when the child had a psychiatric disorder. Gender differences emerged in the interactions of adolescent daughter dyads who were more critical when mothers clearly suffered from a major depressive disorder. A report on group therapy for adult daughters of mentally ill mothers found that the daughters hated themselves and their mothers (Williams, 1998). Another common feature shared by these daughters was their perception of themselves as troubled. In short, illness in the child or mother created communication problems of which the outcome can only be harmful and long-lasting.

The final study in this section investigated maternal depression and coping with adolescent children (Klines-Dougan and Bolger, 1998). An interesting finding was the similar coping styles in the offspring of both well and depressed mothers. However, there were a few important differences. The coping style of the adolescent children was weakly related to the mother's current psychological state and the type of depressive symptoms she exhibited. Children of depressed mothers distanced themselves more from their mothers than did the children of well parents. This study confirms the interactional nature of family relationships. As a result of depression mothers tend to isolate themselves, and the older children respond to that by distancing themselves even further (see the case example of Mrs. Dale). Distress is then enhanced for all.

Depression in the mother has many negative consequences for the children. Obviously, younger children are more at risk than older children. Parental depression has special relevance for us, because many of our pain clinic patients are depressed. The case illustration of Mrs. Dale shows how depression in the mother, who also had a long history of unrelenting headaches, affected her two children quie differently.

CASE OF MRS. DALE

Mrs. Dale, 43 years old, patient for years at a pain clinic, with complaints of unremitting tension-type headache. Married, she had one son (John) and one daughter (Ann). Despite her pain, she worked full-time and managed her domestic affairs quite well. Her husband was a mild-mannered man who depended on his wife greatly and was not very involved in domestic affairs. The children did not present any problems. Mrs. Dale seemed especially attached to her son, her firstborn. The relationship with her daughter was quite good, but apparently this child had a mind of her own, and this led to occasional rifts between daughter and mother. Mr. Dale always sided with his daughter.

This relatively steady family situation came under great strain when Mrs. Dale developed clinical depression. She received immediate psychiatric assessment, and the diagnosis of major depression was confirmed. Her depressive illness lasted nearly four years, during which period the family situation deteriorated significantly. One of her symptoms was prolonged isolation in her bedroom, for days or even weeks. During this isolation, she virtually starved herself, and cried a great deal. She lost her job, and the family situation, particularly the daughter's behavior, took a sharp turn for the worse.

The rest of the family members learned to fend for themselves. At this time Ann was about 12 years old. The first troublesome event was Ann's theft of some article from a neighbor's house which had no particular use to her. She made no serious effort to conceal her crime and was easily found out by her father. He did not make a big issue of it, but had a quiet talk with her. When Mrs. Dale discovered this transgression, she severely chastised Ann, made her return the article, and apologize to the neighbor. This was the beginning of the Ann's "rebellious" behavior.

At this stage, Ann's attitude was defiant. She refused to help with the household chores, ignored her mother completely, and spent almost all her time in her room. Mrs. Dale's behavior toward Ann was inconsistent. John seemed relatively unaffected by his mother's illness. Mr. Dale was beginning to show signs of frustration, which he mainly expressed by silence (passive–aggressive behavior), due to lack of progress in his wife's condition. He remained very sympathetic to Ann.

Over the next two years Ann's behavior worsened. She played truant at school and her work there declined, categorically refused to do any household chores, and stayed out late without permission. What upset Mrs. Dale most was that Ann completely ignored her mother. This drove Mrs. Dale to distraction. She sought professional help for Ann and was told that Ann's behavior, while worrisome, did not suggest any underlying psychiatric problem. She was trying to gain some autonomy and was reacting to her mother's illness. This was small comfort for Mrs. Dale, and only added to her sense of guilt. During her well-phase, Mrs. Dale would be unduly solicitous of Ann, but all her effort to establish communication was rebuffed. This state of affairs lasted some two years, during which time the marital situation worsened to the point that Mrs. Dale even considered separating from her husband.

As Mrs. Dale's depression began to improve over time and she had longer and longer periods free of depression, the entire family situation began to improve, albeit almost imperceptibly. Mrs. Dale became more and more determined to win Ann over. She started sharing with Ann what it was like to be depressed for so long and how hard it must have been for Ann. As Ann approached her fifteenth birthday, the entire situation seemed much improved. Mrs. Dale's depression improved to the point that she was discharged by her psychiatrist. Simultaneously, the intensity and frequency of her headaches declined so that her visits to the pain clinic were reduced.

This case tells a common tale. Ann virtually lost her mother at a very critical point in her development. This loss was of a very complicated nature. Mother was there and not there. Mrs. Dale's depressive illness accounted for much of Ann's distress, and distress it was. Ann was not suffering a psychiatric disorder, nor was she depressed, certainly not in a clinical sense. Some of her behavior could indeed be accounted for by her adolescence. Yet the inconsistency in Mrs. Dale's behavior, her rather elusive illness, Ann's unexpressed fear about her mother's illness, marital conflict, and a caring, but distant and distraught father, put Ann at considerable jeopardy. Happily, as mother's health improved so did Ann's. This case heightens the need for comprehensive individual and family therapy for parents with depression.

PARENTAL DISABILITY

LaMata and associates (1960) investigated eight families where the father was rendered disabled in a trauma of one year's duration or less and the degree of recovery was not above 70% of his former capacity. One significant conclusion was that the children's ages were major determinants of their reaction to parental disablement. The younger children (ages unknown) manifested a variety of psychological and psychophysiological symptoms. The older children were less affected. This paper has clinical, but no research, value.

Buck and Hohnmann (1982) studied 45 children whose fathers had suffered from spinal cord injuries. The children were divided into two groups: those whose fathers were paraplegic and those whose fathers were quadriplegic. The mean age of the children in the paraplegic group was 21; for the quadriplegic, 21.6 years. The inclusion criteria specified the ages of the children to be between 18 and 30, the child had to be two years old or younger when the father was injured, the parents' marriage had to be intact at least until the child was 15 years of age, and the father had to be a veteran. The severity of parental disability and child adjustment were measured on more than 150 variables, which included health patterns, athletic involvement, interpersonal relations, parent–child relations, and personal attitudes.

The study found relatively few relationships between severity of parental disability and children's adjustment. Interesting differences were found between the children of quadriplegics, who reported contact with mental health professionals, and paraplegics, none of whose children had such contacts. The number of children seeking mental health care was very small. The authors urged caution in interpreting the data due to the small sample size, bias for subject selection and reliance on self-reports. However, the study is valuable because it reveals the benign long-term effects of parental disability. Middle-class families with a stable marriage, good income, and no concern about medical costs minimize the negative consequences of parental disability. In a major literature review on parental disability and its effects on children, Buck and Hohmann (1982) concluded that research provided little reliable and valid information due to serious methodological inadequacies and the limited scope of most studies.

More recent studies, with improved methodology, are more promising (Armistead *et al.*, 1995; Worsham *et al.*, 1997). An investigation into the impact of fathers with hemophilia (65 families), approximately 50% of whom were HIV positive, on children (between 3 and 18) found that uncertainty about the fathers' illness predicted anxiety and depression. In addition, children were predictably affected by their mothers' uncertainty, which in turn further contributed to their anxiety (Steele *et al.*, 1997).

PARENTAL CHRONIC PAIN: CASE ILLUSTRATIONS

We begin with two case vignettes to show, at least clinically, some problems children encounter when parents are significantly disabled by pain. We briefly discussed the case of Mr. Bloom in Chapter 2 in relation to unemployment. Recall that this man committed suicide. The emergence of his chronic pain and the behavior that ensued especially after he lost his job had adverse consequences for his children John (19), Mary (15), and James (14). They responded quite differently to their vastly altered circumstances. They lost a friend and confidant in their father. As a result of his pain, Mr. Bloom, described by John as a tyrant, was highly critical of his children, and they were at a loss as to know how to please him. The change in his personality from a caring, albeit authoritarian, father with whom they enjoyed a truly close relationship to that of a tyrant affected each child differently. Mrs. Bloom tried to be a peacemaker but was ineffectual. She generally sided with her husband while feeling powerless with the children.

John "solved" the conflicts by removing himself from the family situation; he stated during the interview that he could no longer tolerate the humiliations heaped on him by his father. He immersed himself in schoolwork and studied late at the college library. Mary became depressed and had a real sense of loss of the closeness she enjoyed with her father. Her schoolwork began to suffer, and she became somewhat of a recluse. Her mother reported that Mary became extremely sensitive and would cry for no apparent reason. James's problems were the most severe. He began using hard drugs, got into bad company, and stayed away from school. These children represented significant behavioral, emotional, and psychological problems of some magnitude. John resorted to a mature way of handling his hurt, but Mary and James were clear victims of their father's chronic pain condition and their mother's inability to protect them.

This case shows the noxious effects of chronic pain, despondency, hopelessness, and depression on children. However, note that many children, especially children in their late teens or older, remain unaffected by family illness. Since most of our patients are in their mid-forties, the children are usually older. It is difficult to bring older children into family assessment situations. We have to rely on parental reports about the children's functioning. It is only when the problems are relatively serious, as with our two cases, that we find ourselves involved.

Our second case illustration is the Dick family. Mrs. Dick is a 39-year-old mother with a history of chronic headache following an automobile accident. Her husband is a professional engineer frequently away from home as a result of his job. They have a son, 14, and a daughter 10. Mrs. Dick's headaches were altogether unpredictable. She might have a whole week without pain and then be rendered totally dysfunctional with severe head pain, which could keep her bedridden for days. She had to leave her lucrative job. Her husband was troubled over how he might find her upon return from business trips. Their son became very withdrawn, and their daughter was increasingly reluctant to leave her mother. The children learned to be quiet round their mother, especially when she was suffering acute pain, but over time it became a pattern. They stopped inviting their friends home lest they should make noise.

The children tried to adapt to their mother's illness, the son by withdrawal and isolation, the daughter with heightened anxiety. These children were not psychiatric victims, neither did they give any evidence of psychopathology, but they were indeed troubled. The kind of distress manifested by them is not generally discussed in the literature, but at a clinical level it is commonly observed. Family intervention is probably the most desirable treatment to counteract the negative consequences encountered by these two children.

LITERATURE REVIEW OF PARENTAL CHRONIC PAIN

We attempt to show that the evidence linking parental chronic pain to their children's health and social problems is at best tenuous. As will be seen, while the research deals with complex problems, yet collectively the findings throw little light on the prevalence of health and psychosocial problems of the children. We first report on general chronic pain syndrome in parents. Next we consider specific pain disorders in parents and their effects on children. Lastly, we examine a few studies that investigated factors that contributed to pain in children.

Dura and Beck (1988) investigated many aspects of family functioning of children of parents with chronic pain or diabetes, and used a control group of healthy parents. Each group comprised seven mothers and seven children. The children of mothers with chronic pain were the most psychologically disturbed, and their family functioning was also the most compromised. Note that the children of chronic pain mothers scored significantly higher on the depression scale, but all three groups of children were in the nondepressed range of that scale. In short, children in all three groups were not depressed. The number of subjects in this study was also a limiting factor. Another study involving 31 children of 19 chronic pain patients found that children of chronic pain fathers were significantly less socially competent than children of chronic pain mothers (Chun *et al.*, 1993). Compared to the control group, children of chronic pain patients had significantly more behavior problems and were less socially competent. However, only a low level of psychopathology was found in both groups.

Roy and associates (1994) investigated the health and well-being of 31 children of 19 patients, 13 females and 6 males, attending a pain clinic. According to the parents, four girls and three boys had problems in the health, emotional/social, and learning difficulties categories. Objectively, however, only three children (less than 10%) were found vulnerable on standard psychological measures. The family profile of these three children was also at variance with the rest of the sample. The negative consequences of parental pain on children were far from evident.

The gender of the parent emerged as an important factor. All three vulnerable patients had mothers who were patients, as were four mothers of the six children with parent-reported problems. The mother's illness is likely to be more disruptive, since the mothers usually continue as homemakers, nurturers, and the contact person with schools and family physicians. Nevertheless, the gender issue was somewhat equivocal as most of the children whose mothers had chronic pain in this sample were not "vulnerable." Mother's illness placing the children at higher risk was confirmed by Dura and Beck (1988) but not confirmed by Chun and associates (1993).

SPECIFIC PAIN DISORDERS IN PARENTS

In an investigation by Rickard (1988) comparing 21 children of parents with CLBP, 21 children with diabetic parents, and 21 children with healthy parents, the children of the CLBP parents were found wanting on several measures, compared with the other two groups. They were more external on the locus of control scale. Teachers reported that there were significantly more complaints, crying, whining, avoiding behaviors, dependency behaviors, absenteeism, and visits to the school nurse than from all other children in this study. Raphael and associates (1990) compared children of 31 patients with Temporo-mandibular joint (TMJ) disorder with 47 controls. Children of TMJ parents reported significantly more illnesses and accidents. A variety of plausible explanations were offered to account for their findings.

Mikail and von Bayer (1990) compared children of headache sufferers with a control group and concluded that the children of headache parents were more prone to be somatically focused, experienced more headaches, and showed greater maladjustment and lower social skills than the children of pain-free controls. A major problem with these findings is that they conducted numerous t-tests and found a low level of significance on many of the associations. The consequences of depression as well as chronic pain are summarized in Table 4.1.

Predictors of Pain in Children

A study by Aaromaa et al., (1998) however, found that in young children suffering from headaches, headache in other family members, especially in the mother, predicted preschool headache in the child. This study was different in

Table 4.1. Some of the Effects of Parental Illness on Children
(as reported in the literature)

Parental depression and children	Maternal Depression and Older Children
a. child adjustment problems	a. obsessiveness
b. parent-child impaired communication	b. more stressors
c. foster care	c. interactional difficulties
d. general psychiatric impairment	d. self-hatred
e. higher psychopathology	e. distancing from mother
f. separation anxiety	
g. somatization	Parental Chronic Pain and Children
h. obsessive traits	a. depression
i. depressive disorders	b. less socially competent
j. phobias	c. emotional/social problems
	d. behavior problems
Maternal Depression and Young Children	e external locus of control
a. infants' social and emotional	f. more illness and accidents
functioning	g. somatization
b. attachment insecurity	
c. Sleep problems	

scope in that the purpose of the investigation was to predict early life factors for headache in children, rather than focusing on the impact of parental headache. Yet it is noteworthy that particularly maternal pain played a complex role in the genesis of pain in the children.

Another study showed that younger children were deprived of parental care during migraine attacks (Smith, 1998). These two studies point up the vulnerability of especially young children to parental head pain. This vulnerability received further support in another investigation of the influence of parental attitudes and illnesses on children with head pain (Gulhati and Minty, 1998). Forty children referred to pediatric neurological service for headache were compared with a matched group of 40 children with recognized pathology, mostly epileptic, for parental illnesses, maternal attitudes, and health beliefs. The finding of most relevance to this discussion was that significant differences were found in the amount of illness experienced by both parents in the headache group. Other factors were the loneliness expressed by the mothers of headache patients, their concern about serious disease in themselves, and reluctance to accept medical reassurance. These last two phenomena are commonly observed in pain clinic populations. The authors noted that family patterns of pain linked with genetic vulnerabilities could partly explain pain in the children, but they cautioned that a link between family stress and tension and the mother's own preoccupation with health could not be overlooked in their decision to refer the child to a specialized clinic.

Another study investigated the relationship between family environment and the functional status of 21 children with juvenile primary fibromyalgia syndrome

(Schanberg *et al.*, 1998). As with previous studies, parental pain history and the family environment correlated with the health status of the children. Parents of these children reported multiple chronic pain conditions, including fibromyalgia.

SUMMARY

We have reviewed three distinct groups of literature. The first group involved a general clinical population with chronic pain and, broadly speaking, failed to produce any convincing evidence of distress in the children of chronic pain sufferers. The second group of studies examined discreet pain conditions in parents and their impact on the children. The results, at best, were mixed. However, there was some suggestion that the children showed more distress and behavioral problems compared to control groups. In the final section, which considered children with a variety of pain problems, the evidence is the most powerful of all. Parental pain, mostly maternal, seemed to be an important variable in predicting health care utilization as well as other kinds of functional and behavioral problems. An amalgam of various factors leads to the following commonsense observation. Maternal ill health, severity of the health problem and associated disability, availability of social support, predisposition of children, and age of the children may all contribute to the health and behavior problems in children of chronic pain patients. A further observation is that the median age of chronic pain patients (early forties and up) suggests that most of their children are likely to be in their teens or older. A common clinical experience is the difficulty we encounter in engaging these children in any therapeutic activities, and quite often patients and their spouses are just as reluctant to involve their children, especially if they are teenagers or older. Nevertheless, as our two case vignettes showed, vigilance is called for in conducting family assessments to probe into the health and well-being of the children.

It would appear that parental ill health has varying levels of consequences on the health and well-being of their offspring. Age of the child, gender of the parent, possibly the gender of the child, severity of the illness, and level of disability are critical factors in predicting the vulnerability of the child (Figure 4.1). Unfortunately, several of the variables listed are either poorly researched or simply have not come under any systematic scrutiny.

Nevertheless, as the case illustrations hopefully exemplify, there exists an information lag between empirical evidence and day-to-day experience of clinicians. Children suffer in different ways. As Rutter pointed out so long ago, many children develop psychological and psychiatric problems in the face of parental illness. Others, as shown by Mrs. Dick's children, do not develop full-blown psychiatric illnesses but suffer emotionally and socially, and if they are left unattended it is conceivable that they may become vulnerable to psychological

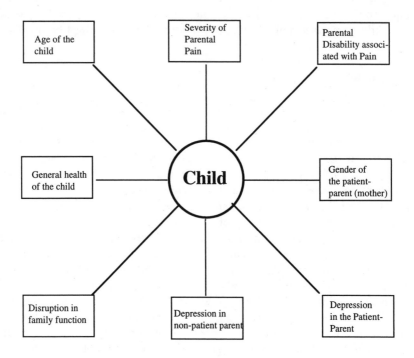

Figure 4.1. Factors influencing impact of parental illness on children.

disorders. As was suggested, family focused intervention may be one way of preventing such an eventuality. Because the average age of chronic pain patients is about 42, their children are often teenagers or older, and, at least in the experience of this author, it is difficult to engage them for therapeutic purposes. Yet many patients, especially with headache, are younger and have young families, and some effort needs to be made to see their children.

Chapter 5

WHAT HAPPENS TO SPOUSES?

INTRODUCTION

In the previous chapter we considered the problem of health and well-being of children of chronic pain sufferers. In this chapter, we turn our attention to the spouses. This is not a new topic. The notion of caregiving to mentally and physically ill persons can be traced to the 1960s, and even earlier. Having a chronically sick person within a family system is more than likely to create demands on the rest of the family members, but most of the extra responsibility is generally borne by the spouse. Considerable evidence of this exists in the chronic pain literature, and research on this subject has multiplied, mainly in relation to the elderly and for caregivers of patients with Alzheimer's disease. Even a casual reading of this literature reveals a wide-ranging research from indicators of health decline among spousal caregivers (Shaw *et al.*, 1997; Vitaliano *et al.*, 1994) to psychological morbidity (Brodaty and Luscombe, 1998) to chronic illness (Kriegsman *et al.*, 1994; Lieberman and Fisher, 1995) and much more.

In a community-based study, involving 1104 white married couples, of the relationship between the husband's health status and his wife's mental health, the results showed that the husband's health, the wife's mental health, and their marital intimacy were highly interrelated (Simonsick, 1993). The husband's health and the quality of marriage were important considerations in improving understanding and treatment of depressive symptoms, low life-satisfaction, and low morale in older women. The availability of close friends had a significant impact on the wife's mental health (Simonsick, 1993). This study has special merit because it involved a large, nonclinical, community-based sample and comprehensive analysis.

Much of this literature has only limited relevance to the trials and tribulations of the spouses of chronic pain sufferers, the reasons being the relatively younger age of the chronic pain population, and a truly different order of problems than those encountered by the caregivers of spouses with organic brain syndromes. Hence, we shall not explore that body of literature.

On the other hand, there is a varied and interesting body of literature dealing with the stress of spousal caregiving for a variety of disorders. We shall examine that literature in some depth because many of the problems are shared by the spouses of chronic pain patients.

Miscellaneous Disorders and Health of Spouses: Spousal distress has come under the scrutiny of researchers in relation to cancer (Rodrigue and Hoffman, 1994), patients in renal failure (Peterson, 1985), brain injury (Krentzer *et al.*, 1994; Linn *et al.*, 1994), multiple sclerosis (Aronson, 1997; O'Brien *et al.*, 1995; Knight *et al.*, 1997;), heart disease (Bookwala and Schulz, 1996; Brady, 1997; Schulz *et al.*, 1997; Thompson *et al.*, 1995), stroke (Morris *et al.*, 1991; Thompson *et al.*, 1990; Thompson *et al.*, 1989) and Parkinson's disease (Carter and Carter, 1994; Hobdell, 1996; Lindgren, 1996; Miller *et al.*, 1996; Walhagen and Brod, 1997). These studies show that caregiving tends to be a hazardous task, albeit varying in the price it exacts. Psychological distress in the spouses of cancer patients (Rodrigue and Hoffman, 1994), loss of sexual activity in the spouses of patients in renal failure (Peterson, 1985), increased depression and long-term health implications for spouses of brain injured partners (Krentzer *et al.*, 1994; Linn *et al.*, 1994) is only a brief list of outcomes.

MULTIPLE SCLEROSIS AND CAREGIVING

A study involving 697 multiple sclerosis (MS) patients (mean age 48 years) and their spouses showed that quality of life for spouses was associated with longer duration of caregiving, moderate or worse symptoms in the patients, and, most strongly, to the patient's current disease course other than when it was stable (Aranson, 1997). In addition, health received the lowest satisfaction rating, while finances received a relatively low satisfaction rating from the caregivers. This study is important because it attempted to measure overall satisfaction with quality of life, and it is evident from the results that the caregivers found their quality of life wanting in many respects.

Another study with MS patients (34) and their spouses (27) sought to identify predictors of general health, mood, family, and life satisfaction for spousal caregivers (O'Brien *et al.*, 1995). The results showed that objective burden, subjective burden, and perceived uncertainty about the illness situation accounted for the largest proportion of variance in the caregivers' general health, mood, and family and life satisfaction. Both studies established that the severity of the illness and the associate demands that emanated from that resulted in poor health and low life satisfaction in the spouses. Uncertainty about the illness is of special interest to us because it tends to plague chronic pain sufferers and their spouses.

HEART DISEASE AND CAREGIVING

A few studies relating to cardiac conditions show various impacts on spousal caregivers. One study investigated a common emotion of caregivers, namely, resentment (Thompson *et al.*, 1995). More resentment was experienced by spouses who felt that their partners were not working toward improved health. This finding is important because its relevance to the spouses of chronic pain patients is evident, since many spouses are not even certain that their partners have a legitimate health problem.

In an investigation of the wives of postmyocardial infarction patients, the results were somewhat optimistic. This study focused on the mental health of wives, 32 to 59 years old, 26 weeks after the infarction. Most spouses were neither depressed nor anxious following their husbands' MI. However, a greater than expected number of women were depressed during the six-month post MI period. A noteworthy fact is that this population was acutely, rather than chronically, ill. In the short term, they had coped well and overcome the danger of death. However, it is intriguing that the level of depression in the wives rose with the passage of time. One possible explanation is that they were now confronted with the reality of living with someone with a defective heart. Realization of this fact alone could contribute to a certain level of apprehension and even depression. This study did not provide any data on the functional state of these patients at six months post-MI. Their level of recovery could be another contributory factor to the presence or absence of spousal depression.

The final study in this section investigated the health effects of caregiving to patients disabled with cardiac disorders (Schulz *et al.*, 1997). This was a large-scale epidemiological investigation. The data showed that about 80% of persons living with a spouse with a disability provided care to their spouses, but only half of the care providers reported mental or physical strain associated with the caregiving. Strain in the spouses was strongly associated with low income and less education. Socioeconomic factors may have measurable negative effects on the health and well-being of the spouse than is generally acknowledged in the research literature on caregiving. If the financial security of the family is compromised, as is often the case with chronic pain, the negative consequences on the spouse are often substantial.

In a rather novel study, Bookwala and Schulz (1996) examined the extent to which one spouse's subjective well-being predicts that of the partner. Subjects were drawn from the Cardiovascular Health Study and involved 1040 spousal pairs. Results showed that one spouse's assessment of well-being and depression predicted the other's well-being even after controlling for known predictors of these outcomes. If the findings of this study can be generalized to other vulnerable groups, then it is conceivable that the relatively high rate of depression in the chronic pain population puts the spousal population at risk for depression. On the other hand, if spouses maintain a sense of well-being, that appears to have a positive effect on the patient.

PARKINSON'S DISEASE AND CAREGIVING

The finding of the Bookwala study received support in an investigation of depression in the caregivers of patients with Parkinson's disease. Subjects included 54 caregivers (friends etc.) of their spouses with Parkinson's and 36 healthy controls (Miller *et al.*, 1996). A patient's depression level emerged as the best predictor of distress in the caregiver, suggesting the importance of treating depression in the patient.

Lindgren (1996) introduced the concept of "chronic sorrow" into her investigation of the spouse–caregivers of patients with Parkinson's. This study, of a very preliminary nature, involved only six patients and four of their spouses. A questionnaire was used to assess chronic sorrow, and two of the four spouses gave evidence of it. What triggered their sorrow included loss of future plans, restricted social life, and inability to travel and participate in hobbies. As a concept, chronic sorrow is useful because it limits the overuse, and sometimes misuse, of the diagnosis of depression, especially for individuals in chronically trying circumstances. An added advantage of this concept is that it does not unnecessarily label persons with a psychiatric diagnosis.

The final study addressed the critical issue of control that patients and spouses encounter in the face of chronic disease, such as Parkinson's (Walhagen and Brod, 1997). Subjects included 101 patients and 45 spouse–caregivers. Perceived control over symptoms was significantly associated with patient well-being, caregiver well-being, and reduced caregiver burden. However, no association was found between the more complex notion of perceived control over disease progression and the foregoing factors. In other words, patients and spouses alike share a certain amount of helplessness in their perception of the course that the disease might take. On the basis of this study, symptom management appears to have a crucial role in maintaining a sense of mastery and control in patients and spouses.

SUMMARY

Even this brief review of the caregiving literature provides an insight into the richness and variety of the topic. Apart from the obvious and more pronounced reaction to caregiving, such as depression, we begin to appreciate some of the lesser known effects such as chronic sorrow, anger, hostility, and a contagion effect, where the mood and outlook of one spouse is reflected in the other. Loss, sadness, and helplessness are some of the other responses noted. We attempt to show in the following section that tension in the spouse of chronic pain sufferers has many different sources, and if we learn anything from the broader literature on caregiving it is that focusing on major emotional and psychological consequences must not occur to the exclusion of less dramatic, but no less trying, consequences of caregiving.

Age, gender, social support, degree of disability, and socioeconomic variables all determine vulnerability of caregivers. To state the obvious, the quality and quantity of caregiving is quite different for a 75-year-old man with a moderate level of Alzheimer's disease than for a man of 50 with chronic heart failure. In addition, although caregiving research is noteworthy for its richness, there appears to be a singular lack of concern with solutions to reducing the risk factors. Again, common sense dictates that solutions will vary a great deal from situation to situation. It could range from home care to psychotherapy and many things in between. In the following section we consider a few solutions.

CHRONIC PAIN AND SPOUSAL DISTRESS

Perhaps a prudent point of departure for this chapter will be to explore the various sources of distress in the spouses of chronic pain sufferers. It is important to recognize at the outset that chronic pain syndrome departs from the conditions described in the preceding section in one significant way. The diagnostic problems of chronic pain conditions are legendary. Many patients only have a working diagnosis, whereas others have a diagnosis such as fibromyalgia, which is viewed with suspicion by many health care professionals and simply rejected by others. This problem alone creates a dilemma for the patient and the spouse which must be, if not exclusive, certainly peculiar. Is one sick or not? While the patient is becoming increasingly disabled by pain, health care professionals continue to express doubt about its source. Even today, with vastly increased understanding of chronic pain, psychiatric explanations are often invoked, or worse, the patient is told that there is nothing wrong with him or her. This problem of dismissive attitude was investigated by Benjamin et al., (1992) in a group of 34 caregivers of chronic pain patients. Most caregivers expressed dissatisfaction with their interaction with physicians, they claimed that they had been offered very little information about the causes and treatment and nothing about their role in the management of pain.

This lack of clarity is obviously of great concern to the patient, but it is also a source of confusion, doubt, and uncertainty to the spouses. This problem and its impact on the relationship itself or on the spouse has attracted little research. In this respect Rowat and Knafl's (1985) study remains of paramount importance. In their investigation of distress in 40 spouses of chronic pain sufferers, one of the central findings was the role of uncertainty as a major source of anxiety in the spouses. Uncertainty about the pain condition itself (diagnostic uncertainty), about the day-to-day behavior of the patient, and about the long-term prognosis create incredible pessimism in patients and spouses. Sometimes, as Rowat and Knafl showed, living with this degree of uncertainty led spouses to develop psychiatric illness.

This problem of uncertainty is routinely encountered in clinical practice. The issues are well illustrated by the case of a Mrs. Ellington, who had long history of chronic headache. Her husband had no way of knowing in what state he was likely to find her on his return from work. Sometimes she stayed in bed all day, other times she functioned well, and on still others she would take to bed during the day. Her condition made it impossible for them to accept invitations and/or to make plans for outings to movies and restaurants. Mr. Ellington was totally demoralized by the situation. He had an intellectual appreciation of his wife's medical condition, but the uncertainty of her behavior drove him to distraction, and his work and mood were affected. His concentration, he claimed, was "shot." The problem became so grave in his mind that in conjoint session he even wondered out loud about the limit of his patience and how long this marriage could last.

Spouses who are repeatedly told that their partner's pain is without obvious medical cause often question the degree of disability displayed and, not infrequently, resent the added responsibilities they are forced to assume. In contrast, many spouses become overly solicitous, and the consequences of that have been the subject of much research in recent years. Another point of note is that not only patients affect caregivers, but caregivers, mainly spouses, influence the patient's mood and behavior.

Although the volume of literature on the impact of chronic pain on the spouse is relatively small, it reinforces the reality of distress in these spouses, under diverse manifestations. Depression, other health problems, and general distress and demoralization have all been reported.

Spousal Distress

Spouses of chronic pain patients appear to be most vulnerable to depression (Ahern et al., 1985; Comstock and Hesling, 1976; Flor et al., 1987; Kerns and Turk, 1985; Saarijaervi et al., 1990; Rowat and Knafl, 1985; Shanfield et al., 1979; Schwartz et al., 1991). The actual rate of prevalence of depression is 16%–19% at the low end (Comstock and Hesling, 1976) to 20%–50% at the upper end (Ahern and Follick, 1985; Flor et al., 1987; Kerns and Turk, 1984; Rowat and Knafl, 1985; Schwartz et al., 1991).

It might be instructive to explore the reasons for spousal distress and depression. Even at the low-risk end, a spouse of a chronic pain patient has more than twice the chance of becoming depressed compared to the general population. Perhaps the research has focused too much on depression to the exclusion of all kinds of distress and difficulties experienced by spouses. For that reason, while exploring possible causes for depression, we try to develop an understanding of other kinds of trials and tribulations experienced by spouses. In several studies the patient's emotional distress appears to have a strong bearing on the spouse's level of distress and depression. Unfortunately, the nature of the patient's distress is rarely elaborated on. One way of appreciating the complex nature of this relationship is through a brief case illustration.

The case of Mrs. Elkes shows the extent of adjustment a spouse is subjected to by role changes that occur through illness. Mrs. Elkes' husband suffered chronic low-back pain for a year, and she recounted to us how in this short time her husband sank deeper into the chronic sick role, she had to become father and business manager as well as an assortment of other roles. For the first time in their 20 years of marriage, she was forced to get a job to make ends meet. Mrs. Elkes was a highly resourceful and resilient individual, and was mostly successful in adapting to her situation. Nevertheless, it would not have been surprising if she developed depressive symptoms under her highly stressful circumstances.

Note that role changes which usually result in an unfair burden on the well partner could be construed as a key source of depression and other manifestations of stress. However, Ahern and Follick (1985) found a weak association between patients' functional impairment and spouses' emotional distress. Schwartz and associates (1991) found that a spouse's appraisal of less impact of chronic pain on the family was associated with a patient's report of a more positive outcome. One interpretation of this finding is that if and when the spouses assumed the additional roles and duties discarded by the patient without much complaint, thus avoiding major disruption in family functioning, the patients reported a positive outcome. Much of the literature fails to address this significant problem associated with role changes, which is often the central source of discontent in the spouse. The concept of "burden," which is so prominent in the caregiving literature, is conspicuous by its almost total absence in the pain literature.

Reasons for Spousal Distress

Clinically, a profound sense of loss and an added burden emerge with singular regularity as causes of distress in the spouses. This was demonstrated in a detailed clinical evaluation of 20 CLBP patients and 12 chronic headache patients and their spouses (Roy, 1989).

It was commonly observed that the spouses struggled with much uncertainty in their daily lives. There is often uncertainty about the nature of the problem itself, especially in relation to back pain. With headache, the uncertainty is centered on the unpredictability of a headache episode, which may disable the patient for a time. Uncertainty also surrounds the prognosis. A third uncertainty is the variation in the daily pain and disability of the patient. Living with uncertainty was mentioned by almost every spouse as a cause of distress. Another source of distress recognized by many spouses was their loss of freedom to give expression to their disagreement and feelings of anger. This suppression of negative emotions may partly explain their tendency to depression, demoralization, and even somatization. The third source of stress that we have alluded to was vast changes in the role functioning of the spouse in response to the patient's decreasing responsibilities.

Roles and Responsibilities and Spousal Distress

In a group of 32 spouses distress due to pain in the partner was common (Roy, 1989). What was not so common was clinical depression or any other major psychiatric disorder. As a group they experienced multiple losses and negative life-events. However, only a few spouses, mostly female, suffered more serious psychological, and in rare instances physical, effects. The male spouses responded by withdrawal, physical and/or emotional, or with anger and hostility.

The worst-affected spouses were married to back pain patients. Although very few of these spouses gave evidence of psychopathology, unhappiness with the marriage was pervasive. Emotional hurt, sadness, feelings of rejection, and other negative emotions were easily observable in almost every spouse of back-pain patients. This is not surprising given the propensity of CLBP patients for rapid decompensation from relatively healthy functioning to sometimes a semi-invalid or even an invalid state. In contrast, the spouses of headache patients were far less affected, a plausible explanation for which was that periodic headache caused far less disruption in the family organization or permanent changes in roles. Spouses of headache patients, as a group, were more adaptable, and their reactions to spousal pain were not excessive.

Another study that investigated changes in the role-related domains reported a significant shift of burden on the spouse (Subramanian, 1991). This study investigated marital disruption and its causes in 20 chronic pain patients and their partners. In the domain of social environment, 48% reported moderate to severe problems, 38% reported problems in sexual relations, and 36% in domestic environment. The Psychosocial Adjustment to Illness Scale (PAIS) was used to measure these dimensions.

In relation to the Domestic Environment subscale of PAIS, the problem areas were interference with work and duties around the house, insufficient help with these duties from the family, and problems with family finances. In the domain of Social Environment, leisure activities, family activities, and participation with friends were compromised. When these two dimensions are viewed together, the picture that emerges is one of more responsibilities and worries (especially about money) and less leisure and fun. Another very telling finding of this study was that 60% indicated low expectations of the patients' ever overcoming their disability, perhaps a major source of sadness and despondency. Although this study did not directly address the question of altered roles, the data clearly show a shift of responsibility from the patient to the spouse and the absence of help from other family members. When these facts are combined with the absence of hope of improvement or recovery of the patient, the likelihood of the spouse developing psychological distress or even dysthymia is quite possible.

Added responsibility and loss of hope in the spouses are often observed in clinical practice. These factors, however, do not necessarily contribute to psychiatric morbidity. For example, Mrs. Emery, a 63-year-old woman, suffered severe back pain at the time of her husband's retirement. Their marital situation, already tense, worsened. Mr. Emery's reaction to his wife's deteriorating health was profound indifference. He showed no understanding of her pain and associated disability, except in one remarkable respect. He quietly assumed nearly all his wife's responsibilities and, at a practical level, was very supportive of her. At an emotional level, however, he seemed to be almost totally disengaged. There was no negative effect of the altered situation on him. Perhaps by taking over her responsibilities, he reinforced her sick role and extricated himself from ongoing marital conflict. These types of complex interplay between patient and spouse have eluded research. Research tends to be linear, exploring cause and effect. As this case shows, rarely, if ever, do complex relationships lend themselves to such a direct cause–effect paradigm. Without a doubt many spouses confronted with huge reversals of fortune brought on by chronic pain in a partner become symptomatic.

The case of Mr. Fortier, age 43, is likely to be familiar to clinicians. At work he suffered back and neck injuries. His condition deteriorated rapidly, and in six months this active, pleasant person was reduced to a semi-invalid. His financial situation forced him to sell his home and move in with his wife's parents. Mr. Fortier's state of mind could only be described as hopeless. Mrs. Fortier's condition deteriorated to the point that she could not stop crying. She lost all interest in her surroundings, including her three-year-old daughter. The situation was made even more complex because Mr. Fortier felt totally responsible for his wife's mental condition. Mrs. Fortier was seen by a psychiatrist and diagnosed with depression brought on by her enormous losses. She was placed on antidepressant medication, and the couple engaged in conjoint therapy.

Summary

Reversal of fortune is common among chronic pain patients. From a fully functioning human being to a semi-invalid status is a difficult adjustment. This transition often occurs at great speed, and losses encountered by these patients and families are huge. Everyone in the family becomes a victim. Spouses in particular are probably most vulnerable. Many become depressed, but most do not. Our case illustrations showed that due to dramatic changes brought on by chronic pain a wife was compelled to join the workforce for the first time, an angry husband of a patient was willing to take over family responsibilities, and, confronted with monumental losses, a spouse succumbed to depression. These cases demonstrate the necessity for a comprehensive family evaluation to ascertain the impact of the patient's condition on the members.

SOMATIC RESPONSES

Apart from depression, a body of literature has investigated the emergence of physical symptoms in the spouses of chronic pain patients. Payne and Norfleet (1986), in their review of chronic pain and the family literature, estimated that a staggering 78% of the family members also reported pain complaints. While there is much evidence of shared pain symptoms among parents and children, evidence related to emergence of pain or other somatic symptoms in the spouses of chronic pain patients is scarce. An early association of chronic pain and spousal somatization was reported by Shanfield and associates (1979). The 44 spouses of chronic pain patients scored significantly higher on Symptom Check List (SLC) 90 for somatization, among other factors, than did nonpatient norms. Mohamed and associates (1978) found that the spouses of depressed chronic pain patients were more prone to developing pain problems than were the spouses of depressed, nonpain patients.

In addition, Block (1981), Flor et al., (1987), and Saarijaervi et al., (1988) also reported physical symptoms in the spouses of chronic pain patients. Block (1981) provided evidence that the spouses of chronic pain patients were prone to developing psychophysiological disorders, and, curiously, the greater the degree of marital satisfaction reported by spouses the greater was the risk for developing illness. Flor and associates (1986), in an investigation of 58 male chronic pain patients and their spouses, reported that the physical symptoms in the spouses were related to the patients' marital satisfaction and their lack of commitment to marriage. However, the only significant predictor of spouses' physical symptoms was their depressed mood, which explained 25.7% of the variance. Finally, Saarijaervi and colleagues (1990), in a study of 31 male and 32 female CLBP patients and their spouses, compared the prevalence of musculoskeletal symptoms among other factors. The only critical finding was that female spouses had significantly more musculoskeletal pain symptoms in the neck and shoulders than did male spouses.

We now briefly explore the explanations for somatic symptoms in the spouses. Flor and associates (1987) described their finding of pain symptoms in the spouses as provocative, suggesting that there is no easy explanation for this phenomenon. They suggested that this finding must be viewed as tentative, and since there is little replication of these findings any explanation can only be speculative. Over the years a variety of explanations has been put forth as determinants of pain symptoms in parents and children as well as siblings. In relation to marital partners, there is a clear paucity of plausible explanations for pain and other physical symptoms in the spouses of chronic pain patients. One obvious one is pain that is quite unrelated to spousal pain. Given the commonness of headache and low-back pain, it is more than probable that spouses will share pain symptoms. It is also quite likely that somatic symptoms are one way of expressing disaffection with marriage. Suppression of emotions is generally associated with this phenomenon. Yet another possibility is simply that depressed spouses also have somatic symptoms since they are ubiquitous in clinical depression. Sadly, there is as yet nothing definitive as far as mechanisms are concerned that might explain high prevalence of pain symptoms in the spouses. These are theoretical possibilities, not uncommonly observed in clinical practice.

Anyone working systematically with families in a pain clinic will readily recognize the regularity with which spouses report one kind of distress or another. Headaches and other kinds of physical problems abound. These cases are rarely straightforward. Frequently, complex situations present themselves as with Mrs. Ford, who had a longstanding gastrointestinal problem. In the meantime, her husband developed severe back pain, which brought him to a pain clinic. The emergence of his pain problem led to much disharmony between this couple. They seemed to be in competition with each other as to who was suffering more. His pain behaviors, which included prolonged periods of rest and missing work, were totally unacceptable to his wife. She remained skeptical about his pain and viewed him as irresponsible and lazy. She blamed him for the worsening of her own GI problem. This marriage had a long history of unhappiness. Nevertheless, there was little doubt in her mind that her own pain condition had been made much worse by her husband's back pain.

This case raises some interesting questions: Is it feasible that the husband's idiopathic back pain was some kind of a reaction to his demanding wife? Is it possible that once his back pain set in that they began to compete as to who was sicker? Was an unhappy marriage at the heart of the complications that arose between them? The first two questions, though clinically challenging, are speculative. The suggestion that their bad marriage was made worse with Mr. Ford becoming chronically ill is perhaps the most plausible one.

In another difficult case, Mrs. Dale had a history of chronic pain and depression (see Chapter 4). Mr. Dale responded to the intractable situation with many vague physical symptoms, such as aches and pains, frustration, tiredness, and occasionally insomnia. He never sought medical help. Nothing, however, interfered with his work and his effort to keep his family together, although he was quite concerned for their young daughter. Only rarely did he express doubt about the severity of his wife's illness, and these were mainly related to an absence of hope for her recovery.

Summary

Symptoms of pain and physical problems are commonly observed in the spouses of chronic pain patients. It is reasonable to assume that many of these symptoms are responses to the various stressors in the spouses' environment brought on by the changes in demands associated with many losses. Physical manifestation for psychological distress is not new. It is one way, in the absence of proper channels for expressing negative emotions, to voice one's distress. Open communication between partners is a frequent casualty of chronic pain. At least at a hypothetical level, it is more than plausible that failure to communicate and suppression of emotions will find expression in physical symptoms. Another reality is that the proportion of spouses who are depressed will also have somatic symptoms. Serious health problems, with the exception of depression, directly attributable to spousal chronic pain have not been reported and are rarely seen in clinical practice. As shown in Table 5.1, spousal problems tend to cut across the types of illnesses. Many more problems have been noted in the spouses of chronic pain sufferers than for spouses of patients with other medical conditions.

OTHER KINDS OF SPOUSAL ISSUES

Literature on disparate aspects of pain and spouses includes a spouse "response model" (Burns *et al.*, 1996), spousal lack of life control and patients' negative appraisal of the pain experience (Flor *et al.*, 1987), spouses contributing to patients' depression and anxiety (Kraaimatt *et al.*, 1995; Waltz *et al.*, 1998), and spousal distress related to the pain severity (Revenson and Majerovitz, 1991). Burns and associates (1996) found that a chronic pain patient's expression of hostile anger and, consequently, poor adjustment was in response to infrequent positive and frequent negative spousal responses. But in a novel study by Kraamaat *et al.*, 1995), pain was found to contribute significantly to depression and to anxiety only in subjects living with a spouse. Another study confirmed that negative spousal behavior predicted worse pain outcome in a population of rheumatoid arthritic subjects (Waltz *et al.*, 1998).

Table 5.1. More Common Consequences of Heart Disease, Parkinson's, and
Chronic Pain on the Spouse (as reported in the literature)

Heart disease	Depression Resentment Strain
Parkinson's	Depression Chronic sorrow Helplessness
Chronic pain	Depression Resentment Anxiety Emotional distress Role changes Somatization

Summary

These last three studies show the very complex nature of marital relationships and indirectly explain the reluctance of spouses to express their negative
emotions. There appears to be a serious cost related to open and honest communication between partners. An interesting area of research will be to explore the
emotional cost exacted from spouses for not expressing their negative thoughts
and feelings. In fact, this entire body of research leaves the interactional nature
of spousal relationship unaddressed. The issues of chronic pain leading to various
kinds of spousal distress and of spousal behavior contributing to more pain and
depression in the patient suggest that these problems, when examined in isolation
from each other, have not been incompletely resolved. The clinical merit of these
findings is of necessity limited, because the scope of the research is so very
circumscribed. Couples live in a complex web of give and take, and affect and
influence each other at all times. If chronic pain causes some spouses to develop
depression, then the spousal depression in turn must also have some consequences
for the patients. However, the most noteworthy point is that a relatively small
proportion of spouses actually succumb to illness. What proportion of them
become unhappy and discouraged and demoralized still remains unknown.

A RATHER COMMON TALE

We close this chapter with a case discussion to show the complicated nature
of the impact patients and spouses have on each other—complicated, yet
commonly observed in pain clinic patients and their partners. Our patient, Mrs.

Foster, is 40 years old diagnosed with fibromyalgia and panic disorder. She has been married for 18 years and has two daughters, ages 14 and 6. She has had panic disorder for the past 10 years and fibromyalgia for 4. The combination of child birth and illness forced her to give up her job, and she became a full-time homemaker. She has pervasive sleep disturbance, constant fatigue, and generally low mood.

Her 43-year-old husband is a self-employed tradesman. In their first visit to the clinic, both partners complained much about each other, neither pleased the other. They were full of mutual recrimination and could hardly recall the qualities they admired in each other that led to their marriage. The conversation gradually moved in the direction of the impact, if any, the illness had on the health of Mr. Foster. Before he even pondered the question, Mrs. Foster interjected that his behavior was making her sicker. He was always grumpy, never smiled, never showed any affection for her, and so on. His behavior was making her feel guiltier for not doing her part in managing the family affairs, especially dealing effectively with the kids. He was making her depressed.

He listened to her silently and then responded as follows. He did not think that her illness had made him sick. He had an intellectual appreciation of both her conditions since he had read up on them and was well informed. However, he resented the additional responsibilities he had to assume in running the family. He listed numerous complaints, but avoided answering the question of how his wife's illness affected his well-being. He acknowledged that emotionally he had moved away from his wife, he felt angry with her but rarely expressed it. He also felt despondent, and sometimes was overwhelmed by sadness. Most of all he had a permanent sense of disappointment because his life had not turned out as he had hoped.

Despondent, disappointed, angry, sad, these were the emotions expressed by Mr. Foster. He was definitely not clinically depressed, but his state of mind led to a certain amount of detachment from his wife and children. Mrs. Foster's reaction to his relative withdrawal was more guilt and more criticism of her husband. The cycle of mutual recrimination and unhappiness continued.

Summary

This case is presented for two reasons: (1) Spousal reaction is not always a florid psychiatric or psychological problem, but can be subdued yet pervasive feelings of sadness and disappointment. (2) These feelings generally set off a cyclical pattern of action and reaction which is very hard to break. Also note that depression in the spouse is certainly not uncommon, and the kind of emotional reaction reported by Mr. Foster is frequently reported by the partners. Research to date has virtually ignored these less dramatic spousal responses and the chain reaction that they set off, leading to great marital disharmony.

We have considered the problem of spousal reaction to illnesses, with special attention to spouses of chronic pain patients. Research has almost exclusively focused on depression and its causes in spouses. There is some literature exploring the impact of spousal behavior on the patient. An argument has been developed in this chapter that spouses almost invariably react to spousal chronic pain, which in turn has consequences for the patient. This circular nature of the spousal relationship, ignored in research, is highly important in the treatment of these couples.

Chapter 6

FAMILY INTERVENTION

INTRODUCTION

Chapters 3–5 give credence to the proposition that the families of chronic pain patients are vulnerable to a variety of negative forces that tend to compromise their general family functioning and raise the risk for children and spouses of becoming depressed, isolated, and demoralized. Our knowledge of these families has increased at phenomenal speed, considering so little was known about them even in the 1980s. This proliferation of research into aspects of chronic pain families has simply not been matched by any curiosity as to what some of the more effective therapeutic interventions would be like. The paucity of outcome research for family therapy with chronic pain patients calls for creative approaches to examine this issue. In this chapter we consider the outcome research on depression and family therapy, other kinds of physical disorders and family therapy, and review the clinical literature on family therapy and chronic pain. Some problems of conducting family therapy with this patient group are discussed.

DEPRESSION AND FAMILY THERAPY

Although the actual prevalence of clinical depression in chronic pain patients and their spouses is open to debate, that many of them succumb to depressive illness is undeniable. The social causes of depression is a time-honored topic of research in the psychiatric literature. Klerman and Weissman (1986) note that "depression, regardless of symptom patterns, severity, the presumed biological vulnerability, or personality traits, occurs in a psychosocial and interpersonal context associated with the onset of symptoms is important to the depressed person's recovery and possibly to the prevention of further episodes."

For chronic pain patients and their families, multiple losses are probably the most common shared experience. Loss of health, loss of job, and loss of intimacy, complicated by significant role changes within the family system, create an optimal situation for depression. In addition, depression is capable of causing major disruption in the family system (Gotlibb *et al.*, 1990). A preponderance of marital and family problems in "neurotic" depressive families as opposed to "endogenously" depressed subjects has also been reported (Birtchnell and Kennard, 1983). Prince and Jacobson (1995), in their excellent review of the relationship between depression and marital discord, identified four main areas of investigation:

1. Relationships between marital distress, loss of social support, and depression
2. Evidence pointing to marital distress as a precursor, concomitant, and consequence of depression
3. Patterns of communication and behavior in couples with a depressed spouse
4. Marital functioning as a predictor of treatment response

In other words, there exists a body of knowledge that supports these four areas, providing a rationale for family or couple treatment for depressed patients. Prince and Jacobson (1995) addressed the critical question of which comes first, depression or marital discord, and provide the following advice: "Given the high concordance rates between marital distress and depression, and the link between unresolved marital disputes and recurrence of depressive symptoms, it seems prudent to pursue the clinical utility of couple therapy for depression even if the research question of "Which comes first?" has not yet been answered." Brown and Harris (1978), in their analysis of social causes of depression in women, produced sufficiently convincing data to support that assertion.

Vaughan and Leff (1976) found an association between family stress (Expressed Emotions) and relapse in patients with affective disorders. Chronic pain is not only capable of producing depression in the patient, but, as the preceding chapter revealed, many spouses also develop this distressing condition. There have been dramatic advances in the pharmacological treatment of depression, and family therapy as an adjunct has been used to address the disruptive effects of depression on the family. For chronic pain patients, where in many cases the social factors loom large, pharmacological intervention for depression may be a partial solution. In any event, there are controlled outcome studies which assess the efficacy of family therapy with depressed patients. We now briefly assess those studies.

The actual number of controlled outcome studies is few, but the results are promising. Prince and Jacobson (1995) concluded that couple and family therapy, while showing promise, had many limitations, for example lack of clarity about which subsets of depressed patients were most likely to benefit from this therapy. However, a review of the psychotherapy literature on the treatment of depression, including family therapy, came to the sad conclusion that "to date, none (of the studies) have established efficacy in controlled clinical trials regarding aspects such as hospitalization, recurrences, or suicidal behavior, as medication alone does" (Colom *et al.*, 1998). Evidence exists that although family and couple therapy may not prevent the disease from recurring, they seem able to modify the negative consequences of depression on interpersonal relationships. This is a critical point in the context of chronic pain. As yet there is no known cure for this syndrome, but family therapy and other psychological interventions can make living with chronic pain more tolerable and less challenging.

Three early studies attested to the benefit of conjoint therapy for depressed patients and their spouses (Epstein *et al.*, 1988; Friedman, 1975; McLean *et al.*, 1975). Friedman's study demonstrated that drugs combined with family therapy produced superior results than four other treatment conditions, which included placebo and minimal therapy. Drugs were highly beneficial in reducing the neurovegetative symptoms, and couple therapy helped to ameliorate family task (role) related problems and improved marital interaction. McLean's study was far less sophisticated in design, but also reported significant improvement in an experimental group of 20 depressed subjects who received one hour of conjoint therapy for eight weeks. Twenty patients in the control group received a variety of interventions, but not couple therapy, and two subjects had no treatment at all. Finally, Problem Centered Systems Family Therapy (PCSFT) was used to treat depressed individuals and their family members with the expressed goal of improving recovery from depression by addressing communication, role, problem solving, and affective issues (Epstein *et al.*, 1988). Family therapy was used in conjunction with pharmacotherapy, and the outcome showed that the addition of family therapy considerably improved recovery from depression.

Three more studies have also yielded positive results (Clarkin *et al.*, 1990; Retzer *et al.*, 1991; Waring *et al.*, 1995). The Clarkin study was an in-patient-based study with 29 unipolar and 21 bipolar subjects. The subjects were randomly assigned to standardized hospital treatment and standardized treatment plus family therapy (IFI). Results in both the short term and long term (18 months) showed that the major beneficiaries of IFI were female bipolar depressives; quite surprisingly, unipolar patients achieved better results without benefit of family therapy. Males, on the whole, reacted negatively to family therapy. A case was made by this study to make selective use of family therapy with patients with affective disorder.

Retzer and associates (1991) reported their findings on the effectiveness of systemic family therapy with 20 (10 males and 10 females) subjects with bipolar mood disorder and 10 (5 males and 5 females) subjects with schizoaffective disorder. After a three-year follow-up, relapse rates decreased 76.7%, 67.8% for manic depressives, and 89.8% for schizoaffectives. Their explanation for these dramatic results was that these families were in a perpetual state of struggle with issues of autonomy and victimization and dependency. This study has not been replicated, and the findings, while tantalizing, remain untested.

The final study in this section was conducted by Waring and associates (1995). The subjects were 17 depressed married women who were assigned to marital therapy or a waiting list control group. Couple therapy consisted of 10 sessions designed to enhance marital intimacy. The marital therapy group had a significant reduction in depressive symptomatology on several standardized measures of depression. The authors proposed that marital therapy designed to enhance intimacy may be a viable treatment for women whose depressive symptoms are initiated by the loss of hope of developing a close, confiding relationship.

Summary

This brief incursion into the outcome studies of family and couple therapy with depressed individuals sought to find another kind of justification for using this method of intervention, mainly as an adjunct, for treating depressed chronic pain patients and their families. The rationale for couple and family therapy is found in a significant body of literature that shows the far-reaching consequences of depression on marriage and family (Brown and Harris, 1978; Prince and Jacobson, 1995). The Waring study is of special interest because it addressed one of the fundamental problems—loss of intimacy—frequently encountered among chronic pain couples. The Retzer study is also relevant to our population because it dealt with issues of autonomy and dependency, again not an uncommon problem in chronic pain families. The Epstein study with its focus on complex areas of family functioning is instructive, since many chronic pain families encounter difficulties in similar dimensions of family functioning (Roy, 1989). In addition to the patients, the spouses of chronic pain patients often struggle with problems of dependency, autonomy, and intimacy. That fact strengthens the argument in favor of considering family or couple therapy.

PHYSICAL ILLNESS AND FAMILY THERAPY

Family therapy outcome studies with medical conditions are a neglected area of research. Two major reviews on this topic reached more or less the same conclusion—that the actual quantity of outcome studies of systemic family therapy with medical and psychosomatic conditions is truly meager (Campbell and Patterson, 1995; Roy and Frankel, 1995). Although anecdotal and clinical descriptions of the use and value of family therapy with a whole host of medical illnesses abound, there is little solid evidence that family therapy has any intrinsic value as an adjunct in the overall treatment of, for instance, rheumatoid arthritis, diabetes, coronary artery disease, or any other chronic disorders (Roy, 1990).

Cancer is an exception, since a few family-oriented outcome studies have been reported and will be presently discussed. The rationale for family therapy with medical disorders is twofold: (1) the influence of family interactions in the development and maintenance of disease or illness behavior; and (2) rectifying the disruption caused by illness in a family system. The role of the family in the etiology of medical illness is almost completely unproven, whereas the role of family members in encouraging and perpetuating illness behavior is not without foundation. Family therapy as a means to counteract the upheaval caused by illness in families is perhaps, at the very least, comprehensible even at a common-sense level. Sadly, however, research in that regard is also limited. Nevertheless, we presently review that literature. Because of the paucity of relevant literature, we include a brief discussion of family-oriented approaches in addition to traditional family therapy.

Family-Oriented Approaches

Over the years several novel approaches have been used when working with families of cancer patients (Goldberg and Wood, 1985; Heinrich and Schag, 1985; Herzoff, 1979; Plant et al., 1987; Theorell et al., 1987). The following three studies had control groups. Theorell and associates (1987) investigated the effects of group intervention for close female relatives of cancer patients. The treatment group and control group each had 36 subjects with mean ages of 52 and 51, respectively. Treatment consisted of psychosocial intervention, information, and medical treatment. Outcome measures included measures of psychiatric symptoms, severity of patient's illness, and measures of cortisol and prolactin levels. Blood samples were obtained monthly. Outcome was based on the relatives who experienced death of the family members. This sample comprised 18 treatment subjects and 17 control subjects. At posttreatment, the prolactin levels were lower in the treatment group. At the time of the patients' death the cortisol level was significantly higher in the treatment group. In addition, the treatment group had significantly lower levels of mental exhaustion following the death of a family member.

Goldberg and Wood (1985) studied lung cancer patients whose spouses were offered interpersonal psychotherapy. Outcome failed to show any significant differences between treatment and control groups on various psychological measures. This study raised the possibility that interpersonal problems cannot be significantly reduced or eliminated if all parties involved are not participants in the therapeutic process.

The third study was reported by Heinrich and Schag (1985). They implemented a couple group therapy program to enhance management of stress and activity in a group of cancer patients. Twenty-six patients and 25 spouses participated in the treatment, and 25 patients were assigned to the control group. The treatment component was a six-week cognitive–behavioral structured small group program. Each session lasted two hours. The objectives of the therapy were to educate the patients and spouses about cancer and to teach specific skills for managing daily stresses. The results showed that the information aspect of treatment increased participants' knowledge of cancer and their coping skills. The control group did not show any such improvement. In contrast, over time both groups became better adjusted on psychosocial adjustment. At the two-month follow-up the treatment group continued to express a high level of satisfaction and were actively using the techniques for stress reduction.

Family Therapy

A study of the efficacy of couple therapy with 20 mastectomy patients and their spouses was reported by Christensen (1983). They received four weeks of structured couple intervention, but the control group did not. The goal of intervention was to improve the couple's relationships, communication, and self-esteem. The results showed significantly reduced depression in the patient, increased sexual satisfaction for both partners, and reduced emotional discomfort in both partners.

One other controlled study investigated the efficacy of intervention to improve communication in 20 hypertensive patients and their spouses (Ewart *et al.*, 1984). Compared to the controls, these couples showed less hostility, fewer combative behaviors, and a significant reduction in systolic blood pressure. However, the intervention was more of an educational nature than actual marital therapy.

Summary

These three diverse family-oriented therapy interventions for relatives, spouses, and friends of cancer patients at least show that these methods can potentially reduce distress and help improve the quality of family life. It will be an error of judgment to make any greater claim. Also note that cancer has attracted a little more attention than any other medical condition for family-oriented approaches. These novel methods have yet to make their way into the treatment of chronic pain sufferers and their families. As the review shows, controlled trials of family therapy for chronic adult illnesses are virtually nonexistent. Another observation is that several major reviews on outcome of family therapy were reported in 1995, and in the last five years nothing has changed. Nevertheless, the findings of actual family therapy and family-oriented therapy are still cause for restrained optimism.

CHRONIC PAIN AND FAMILY THERAPY

In this section we examine clinical reports on the application of family therapy to the chronic pain population, and provide a case illustration to show the value of this activity. Chapters 3–5 gave ample evidence that chronic pain families face many critical issues, and the justification for family intervention is derived from the facts elucidated in those chapters. In our discussion of cases, we show some of the limitations of family therapy. We start with a case that illustrates some problems of role functioning and communication and the couple therapy that was applied.

A SIMPLE CASE?

Mrs. Good, 29, was referred to a pain clinic by her neurologist. She had suffered from a combination of muscle contraction and migraine headaches of many years duration, and her health had deteriorated. Although she disliked taking medication, she was consuming analgesics in ever-increasing amounts. The neurologist speculated that other issues, which were not self-evident, were affecting her behavior. In spite of our request to bring her spouse for the first interview, as was the custom of the clinic, she arrived alone. She was smartly dressed and highly articulate. She gave no external sign of distress or discomfort and physically appeared in good health. She confirmed the neurologist's concern that her headaches had worsened and, because she was ingesting a vast quantity of narcotic analgesics, she feared becoming an addict.

She was quite puzzled over the sudden deterioration of her condition, but denied any feelings of depression or sadness. She did mention that she was recently placed on anti-depressant medication by her family physician. She was unsure of the purpose of this medication and, perhaps correctly, thought of it as another analgesic.

Having reviewed her headache condition, we probed her social situation. Two close members of her extended family who were very close to her had recently died. She had just returned to a university after several years to finish her degree. Her husband was totally preoccupied with his Ph.D. thesis. The couple had two children, age 5 and 3.

Mrs. Good's return to school had upset the entire family arrangement. She encountered domestic conflicts and serious issues of child care, which remained unexpressed. She insisted on maintaining all her household responsibilities lest her husband's academic progress be hampered. In brief, we told her she was doing too much, was sad, and had no one to share with. She was told to bring her husband for the following session.

The problems facing Mrs. Good seemed obvious. Unresolved grief, a self-absorbed husband, enormous domestic responsibilities, and perhaps very poor timing on her part to return to school. Not falling academically too far behind her husband was a plausible concern of hers. The absence of confidantes was also striking. Her husband was simply unavailable, or she chose not to burden him with her mounting anxieties and sadness, or worse he was indifferent and uncaring. Under those circumstances, exacerbation of her headache was not altogether inexplicable.

Treatment Issues

Mr. and Mrs. Good kept the next appointment. Mr. Good was hesitant and did not say much during the early part of the interview. Mrs. Good spoke mainly about how hard her husband worked. Some of the recent changes in the family organization were discussed. Mr. Good was apparently concerned about his wife going back to school while she had so much responsibility, but he was less than emphatic because he did not want to interfere with his wife's desire to finish her degree. He was very conscious of his relative disengagement from the family, especially over the past several months. He expressed a certain amount of guilt, but reassured his wife that the situation was short-lived. She, on her part, expressed her complete support for what he was doing. In other words, they were both agreeing to maintain the status quo.

The therapy that ensued over the next few sessions was mainly focused on communication and role-related issues. Mrs. Good's headaches were rarely mentioned throughout this process. The couple was encouraged to discuss their respective roles, especially sharing child care responsibilities, and consider how they could be more effective in performing those roles. They were asked to explore ways of supporting each other and be more open in their communication. Mrs. Good felt constrained in sharing her feelings in view of her husband's heavy load, and Mr. Good failed to discourage her from going back to school at a stressful time in their lives. In therapy, they made rapid progress. Mrs. Good decided to switch to evening courses, when Mr. Good assumed child care responsibilities. They also gave evidence of being more open about their desire to be less protective of each other and more willing to share their feelings. At the six-month review, at which time she was relatively pain free and the family situation continued to be relatively stable, Mrs. Good was discharged from the clinic.

Summary

This case was chosen to show that exacerbation of pain can, at least in part, be brought on by changes in family organization. This couple found themselves in a bind, both protective of each other. Arguably, Mrs. Good's worsening headache had an important message value. It was through her pain that she conveyed the untenable nature of her family situation. Returning to school at a time when her husband was unavailable further destabilized the situation. More pain was the outcome. Nevertheless, once this couple was given a platform to discuss the issues openly and candidly, not only was the level of intimacy between them enhanced, but Mrs. Good's headaches showed signs of improvement. It must be recognized that this marriage was basically healthy, but circumstances had contributed to considerable strain on the family system, rendering it quite problematic. In many ways it was a simple case. This young family functioned well until Mr. Good's withdrawal from the family. The burden was too great for Mrs. Wood. She sought help for a medical problem. Fortunately, the neurologist, and, subsequently, the pain clinic professionals were able to reformulate the problem in terms of the changes in her family situation.

FAMILY THERAPY AND CHRONIC PAIN LITERATURE

In the absence of outcome literature, we shall confine ourselves to an exploration of the various models of family and couple therapy that have been used to work with this population. Strategic and structural models of family therapy subscribe to the etiologic significance of family dynamics in the development of pain symptoms. It must be emphasized that the evidence for that claim is solely anecdotal. Strategic family therapy is based on the assumption that faulty communication usually results in family dysfunction and can induce pain symptoms.

Strategic Family Therapy

Reports of strategic family therapy to treat pain symptoms are very few. Although numerous allusions to the problem of pain can be found in Haley's writing, mostly demonstrating the message value of pain, he described only one case, that of abdominal pain in a woman which was resolved by some very ingenious and strategic maneuvers (Haley, 1973). Madanes (1981) described a case of a little boy with headache where the pain was reframed to connote parental discord. Successful treatment of parental problems resolved the child's headache. Obviously strategic family therapy with its emphasis on the meaning of pain has limited application in the treatment of chronic pain. On the other hand, as in Mrs. Good's case, it would be hard to deny that pain, which always conveys distress, may also convey other kinds of messages.

Structural Family Therapy

Reports of structural family therapy to treat pain problems are also few and far between. Much of this work was conducted by Minuchin's group during the 1970s at the Philadelphia Child Guidance Clinic. Other than a case report on a severe headache and a treatment report on the efficacy of structural family therapy in treating 10 children with abdominal pain, followed by another study involving 19 children with abdominal pain, and their families, application of this model to the adult population is limited (Koch *et al.*, 1974; Liebman *et al.*, 1976; Berger *et al.*, 1977). These studies did not have control groups and reported a very high rate of successful outcome.

Kunzer (1986) suggested that structural family therapy can "aid pain control treatment by changing transactional patterns of enmeshment, overprotectiveness, rigidity, and lack of conflict resolution that often characterize families with a member with chronic pain." The problem with this assertion is that it is not backed by research. To what extent chronic pain families share the characteristics outlined by Kunzer remains a matter of speculation. Saarijaervi and associates (1989) developed a time-limited, five-session couple therapy, based on a structural model, to investigate its effectiveness with 29 patients with CLBP and their partners. Success was limited, and the study lacked a control group. However, as far as is known, this was the first attempt to systematically apply structural family therapy to treat a chronic pain problem in an adult population.

Strategic and structural family therapies do not as yet have definitive and demonstrated value in treating chronic pain conditions. On the other hand, strategic family therapy enables a therapist to ask the fundamental question: What is the meaning of the patient's pain? What is the patient trying to convey through pain? This contribution is not insignificant. Structural family therapy enables the therapist to examine the negative changes in the family organization as a consequence of chronic pain which may be amenable to successful intervention.

Problem-Centered Systems Family Therapy

This model of family therapy to treat chronic pain families has been almost exclusively reported by Roy, and eventually culminated in a book (Roy, 1989). In addition to showing its efficacy at a clinical level, Roy also reported on its shortcomings. The strength of this model is its assessment tool known as the McMaster Model of Family Functioning (MMFF). The MMFF measures family functioning along the dimensions of problem solving, role, communication, affective responsiveness, affective involvement, behavior control, and a general area. This model makes no etiological claim, but rather is designed to explore the impact of illness and other situations on the family system.

To date there are no outcome studies related to chronic pain that use this model. Roy (1989) reported a preliminary clinical investigation using this model of therapy with eight headache patients and their partners who completed this treatment. They were compared with eight other couples who dropped out. One tentative conclusion was that couples who completed therapy were more stable in their relationship, and the problem of pain had limited negative consequences for them. A combination of recent life-events and pain brought them to the clinic.

In contrast, marital strife was evident in the dropout group. This was a preliminary study which generated some interesting hypothesis.

Roy (1989) also described the lives of 32 patients (20 with headache and 12 with back pain) and their families. Family therapy based on PCSFT was found useful by 16 couples in the headache group and only four couples in the back-pain group. This was by no means a scientific study of family therapy outcome, but it is one of the most comprehensive of its kind. The whole field awaits well-designed control studies to determine the efficacy of family therapy for chronic pain.

In addition, reports promoting the use of family therapy with the chronic pain population exist (Hudgens, 1979; Merskey and Magni, 1990; Kerns and Payne, 1996; Rueveni, 1990, 1995; Saarijarevi, 1992; Watson *et al.*, 1992). They acknowledge the value of not only the critical role that families could play in the recovery of the patient but also the enormous pressure that families experience with a chronic pain patient. Family therapy is justifiable on both counts.

In the remainder of this chapter we consider some common problems encountered in family therapy with the chronic pain population, primarily through case illustrations. Recall that Mrs. Good failed to bring her husband to the initial session. Unfortunately, that appears to be the rule. In our experience we encounter an extraordinary level of resistance to engage the whole family or even the partners. For example, Mrs. Graham, 35 years old, with a prolonged history of severe head and back pains, revealed serious difficulties in almost every aspect of her life, such as financial problems and the strain of working and caring for her family (husband and two preteen children). It was clear that she received no help from her husband and children. Her husband had a very bad temper and at one time was a heavy gambler, which caused untold misery for Mrs. Graham.

Mrs. Graham needed little persuasion to bring her husband. Mr. Graham, however, came to one session grudgingly. He was persuaded that his wife created her own misfortune. She was too tight-fisted with money, and he did not know what to make of her health. Doctors were unsure about the cause of her pain. He thought she should try harder and just get on. His life was demanding with work and his union activities, and he really had no time for domestic activities. He was emphatic, though, that he never neglected his children. As for ongoing family counseling, he failed to see any value in it. His attitude could be summarized as follows: "If she has a health problem, fix it, and then we can get on with our lives. Talking about it won't help." Note that, in many cases, both partners refuse couple therapy.

The reasons for refusing couple or family therapy are many. Nevertheless, for many patients in search of a cure for their pain affliction, any method of treatment that deviates from their conception of medical intervention is all too readily rejected. Many patients challenge the value of family therapy since they believe it is not likely to solve their pain problem. For some couples pain and disability can resolve long-standing conflicts, and they have little or no investment in family or other kind of psychotherapy. We mention the case of Mr. and Mrs. Green. Mr. Green, 42, an immigrant from South Asia, had a humble job, which was a source of great tension between him and his wife. She accused him of lack of ambition and drive. He quietly accepted her criticisms, but did not seek a better job.

As a result of a work-related accident, Mr. Green developed severe chronic back and neck pain. Mrs. Green became his chief advocate with the medical community, workers compensation board, and others, and Mr. Green was happy to remain in the background. His disability removed the pressure on him to better himself, and Mrs. Green was determined to prove his disability to the world. He could no longer work, which was not only acceptable to Mrs. Green, but acknowledged vehemently. The accident released them from their mutual struggle. For them family or couple therapy was not even a consideration. This kind of complex family dynamics is far from revealing and has the outward appearance of great adaptation on the part of the patient and great understanding on the part of the spouse. These patients can pose a serious challenge to rehabilitation.

Our final case illustrates a successful couple therapy. Mr. Grindley, 31 years old had a lifelong history of muscle contraction headache. His pain worsened just before his marriage, and he sought medical help. His referring neurologist described him as a pleasant fellow who seemed unresponsive to treatment. Mr. Grindley was willing to accept psychological help. He came with his wife to the first session. Shy people, it took a couple of sessions for them to be forthright. Mr. Grindley described himself as a loner. He displayed an enormous sense of guilt and remorse at his headaches, especially because they got very bad before his marriage. He was convinced that he had let his wife down. She felt left out and sad about their lack of closeness and intimacy, which was attributed to the headaches. Mr. Grindley acknowledged that he had a great deal of apprehension and felt overwhelmed by his marital responsibilities and added pressure at work. His wife's response was further withdrawal from him.

The therapy focused on promoting intimacy between the couple, without the headache problems. They readily agreed that marriage was a greater challenge than they had anticipated. Mr. Grindley expressed his fear of failing in this relationship and not living up to his wife's expectation. She had similar fears and apprehensions. A plan to promote togetherness without undue pressure was developed. Mr. Grindley was encouraged to inform his wife of his headaches and try not to withdraw from her. Mrs. Grindley was urged to be less willing to accept his retreating behavior. Above all they began to share their fear of letting each other down. They were encouraged to engage in simple enjoyable tasks, such as walking, and to make plans for movies, concerts, etc. This couple was seen for nine sessions over four months. At the last session, Mr. Grindley's headaches had become more manageable and the marital situation was significantly improved.

One way of understanding this case is from the perspective of the difficulties generally encountered by families in formation. Such time can be particularly challenging in a relationship. Two individuals bring their experiences and expectations, which may conflict, into the marriage. Mr. Grindley's fear of closeness was the central problem. He feared marriage and his ability to be a satisfactory partner. More pain and guilt were the consequences. Mrs. Grindley responded by withdrawal and felt responsible for contributing to her husband's pain. Mostly she felt rejected and sad. The entire situation was further complicated by worsening headache, which seemed to be directly related to Mr. Grindley's anxiety about marriage.

Summary

This last case may not be truly typical of the pain clinic population. Mr. Grindley was employed and, in many respects, a fully functioning human being. Unlike many pain clinic patients, he was not disabled by his pain. That therapy was successful with this couple is not surprising. At a purely hypothetical level, it is reasonable to surmise that relatively-well-functioning patients and spouses who are aware of family problems may be best suited for couple or family therapy.

However, there is no guideline for clinicians to follow. Common sense dictates that many stable marriages are strained by chronic pain, and these individuals are generally more amenable to family therapy. As noted earlier, if one or both members are involved in maintaining the patient's sick-role, the chances of success for even engaging these couples appears to be slim. The question asked by many family members, "Is family therapy going to help with the pain?" must be answered directly and honestly. No, family therapy is not likely to have any effect on pain, but it might enable the family to cope more effectively with changes brought on by chronic illness. It is an optimistic message. Unfortunately, it is not always heard that way by families.

Recall that a handful of controlled studies do show the value of family-oriented therapy. They provide, albeit indirect, justification for family therapy with a medically ill population. Given the relative pervasiveness of family problems in the chronic pain population, perhaps greater attention needs to be paid to family treatment outcome research. In the meantime family therapy, remains largely a marginal clinical activity in many, if not most, pain clinics.

Chapter 7

THE NATURE OF SOCIAL SUPPORT

INTRODUCTION

In his famous paper Gerald Caplan (1981) proclaimed the power of social support to reduce an individual's vulnerability to mental and physical illness (Figure 7.1). Even then there was sufficient empirical support for that proposition. Since then, however, there has been a veritable explosion of research, much of it confirming the buffering power of social support against morbidity (Table 7.1). We confine ourselves to the most recent literature.

It is now generally accepted and is supported by research literature, that social support acts as a buffer against the vicissitudes of life, including morbidity. In simple terms, intimate and reciprocal relationships seemingly have the power of protecting individuals from succumbing to illness, or, coping with it more effectively. This proposition has been generally affirmed in many studies involving diverse populations and diverse situations (Koniarek and Dudek, 1996; Penninx, et. al., 1997; Kriegsman et al., 1997; Ystgaard et al., 1999).

The debate about social support in the chronic pain literature has more recently centered on the merit of spousal support, which tends to reinforce pain behaviors. That debate has been extensively examined by Thomas and Roy (1999). We avoid that debate and instead focus on two aspects of social support. First, the value of social support in coping with chronic pain conditions, and to that end we conduct a selected review of recent empirical literature. Second, we explore the clinical and therapeutic value of social support through case illustrations.

RHEUMATOID ARTHRITIS AND SOCIAL SUPPORT

The social support literature in relation to rheumatoid arthritis (RA) falls into several categories. The most dominant literature, however, pertains to the buffering power of social support against depression and psychological distress in persons with RA (Bar-Tal, 1994; Evers et al., 1997; Goodenow et al., 1990;

87

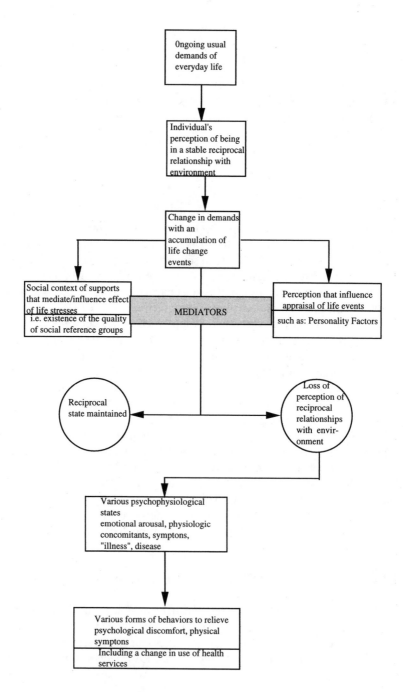

Figure 7.1. Social support and personality factors as mediators of stress.

Table 7.1. Examples of Support Systems

Informal systems	Semiformal systems	Formal systems
Spouses/partners	Workplace	Medical services
Children	Church	WCB
Parents	Volunteer organization	Insurance companies
Friends/relatives	Family physician	Legal systems
Close friends		Canada pensions
Neighbors		

Lambert *et al.*, 1989; Parker and Wright, 1997; Scharloo *et al.*, 1998). Other research shows a weak relationship or an absence of the buffering effect of social support. Only a few publications explore the value of social support in arthritic patients and their general functioning (Manne and Zaruta, 1989; Reisine and Fifield, 1995; Weinberger *et al.*, 1990).

DEPRESSION, PSYCHOLOGICAL DISTRESS, AND SOCIAL SUPPORT

In a literature review on depression and RA, lack of social support was reported as highly significant in the etiology of depression in this patient population (Creed and Ash, 1992). Although the studies in this section are varied in aim and scope, they confirm the value of social support in mitigating depression in arthritic subjects. We only present a selected review of the most current literature. In a prospective study Brown and associates (1989) interviewed 129 subjects with rheumatoid arthritis and rated their satisfaction with several aspects of social support. Their findings confirmed that (1) disruptions in relationships with actual and potential support providers constituted a source of stress; (2) the illness had strengthened the valued relationship; and (3) the relation between support satisfaction and psychosocial adjustment increased as a function of a subject's level of disability. This last finding suggested a stress-buffering effect of support.

The following studies furnished more direct evidence of the buffering power of social support. Fitzpatrick and associates (1988) investigated social relationships in 158 patients with RA. They studied the effects of severity of disease activity and of disability on social relationships. Intimate relationships were less affected than diffuse relationships, such as with friends. The pivotal finding was that the greater the score on social relationships, the more favorable were their scores for depression on the Beck Depression Scale. The social relationships, however, did not buffer the more direct impact of RA. The question is, did the absence of depression result in better overall functioning in spite of the disease state?

The following study explored the issue of the demands of paid work and family work in 262 women with RA. The subjects reported high levels of psychological demands in both family and paid work. High autonomy in family work had a mediating effect on the family demands. The most critical finding of this study was that having higher social support reduced the effects of work demands on depressive symptoms.

A study that has direct relevance to the issue of pain investigated whether support buffered the adverse effects of arthritic pain or resulted in a decrease in pain severity regardless of pain levels in 233 patients with RA. The results were complex. On the one hand, patients who reported higher satisfaction with their social support when experiencing a higher level of pain were less likely to be depressed than patients who did not receive such support. On the other hand, social support did not have any moderating effect on the pain itself. Causal modeling revealed that pain and social support contributed to a change in depression over two six-month intervals.

In a straightforward Dutch study, Doeglas and associates (1994) investigated the direct and moderating effect of social support on the association between social disability and psychological well-being in 54 RA patients. Receiving greater daily social support positively related to greater psychological well-being. People receiving more social companionship were less depressed.

The following reports focus on the question of spousal social support and RA patients. Arguably, spousal support is probably the most critical of all social support in terms of intimacy and the constancy factor. The issue of intimacy is evident, and constancy implies availability of support on a consistent and regular basis. The quality of the marital relationship is unquestionably of critical import. This quality issue was addressed by Manne and Zaruta (1989) in their investigation of spouse criticism and its effects on psychological adjustment among 103 women with RA. Predictably, patient adjustment was significantly related to spousal attitude: the more critical the spouse, the more maladaptive was the behavior displayed by patients. When the spouse was perceived as supportive, patients engaged in more adaptive coping.

The fact that social support does not necessarily translate into low or no depression was reported in a study of 64 married patients (Schiaffino and Revenson, 1995). Subjects who did not experience a sense of challenge in response to a diagnosis of RA had the lowest level of depression when they received higher positive support from their spouses. However, the situation changed as a sense of challenge resulted in elevated depression in spite of greater positive support. It appears that heightened anxiety may not be amenable to support, but how social support might have contributed to higher depression is far from evident.

Social support is naturally contingent upon the ability to provide such support. On the other hand, it is possible that the spouse may fall prey to depression and ill health due to chronic illness in the partner. Revenson and Majerovitz

(1991) investigated the relationship between depression and the support spouses received from their RA partners and social network. Greater marital adjustment was related to lower symptoms of depression. However, when the disease was more severe, and presumably the patient support was compromised, spouses with greater network support still experienced fewer depressive symptoms. This study provided at least partial support for the network stress-buffering model.

The final study in this section examined marital quality and its effects on individual variability in pain severity in 136 Dutch and 98 German subjects with RA (Waltz et al., 1998). Patient reports of negative spouse behavior and baseline depression predicted a worse pain outcome, and this association remained significant in analyses controlling for baseline pain. Second, daily emotional support and positive social life domains influenced the outcome. Finally, the absence of strong social ties was the component of loneliness linked to pain.

The Questionable Value of Social Support

While the preceding review has affirmed the intrinsic merit of social support in relation to RA, the following section considers the research literature, albeit rather scanty, that raises questions about the value of such support. That social support of a spouse is no guarantee for better mental health was demonstrated in a study of female RA patients, 22 of whom were never married, 127 were living with a spouse, and 53 were widowed or divorced. No significant differences were found in depression and anxiety between the never-married group and the currently married subjects (Kraaimaat et al., 1995). Widowed or divorced women had less potential support and more depression and anxiety than subjects who were never married or who were living with a spouse. The widowed or divorced patients had lower income than the other groups. Less potential support was related to more anxiety. One curious finding was that pain emerged as a significant factor contributing to depression and anxiety only in subjects living with a spouse. This finding is perplexing because it contradicts the trend that affirms the power of social and emotional support as a buffer against depression and other psychological problems. Without controlling for a whole host of factors related to marital functioning, which this study did not, this finding must be viewed as tentative.

That the power of social support as a buffer can be compromised by personality factors was shown in a study involving 138 female patients with RA (Fryand et al., 1997). They found that the effect of emotional support on mental health was spurious and dependent on personality traits. The total effect of social support was moderate compared to a strong influence of neuroticism. This study raises the issue of patient capacity to derive the full benefit from social support, and the suggestion is that certain kinds of personality traits tends to neutralize or at least lessen the potential benefits of emotional support.

Roberts and associates (1996) investigated the value of different types of social support (tangible, emotional, informational and integrative) in a group of 27 men and 32 women with arthritis. One important finding was that only low tangible support attenuated the negative effects of functional impairment on depression. Other types of support either failed to have any effect at all or worsened the deleterious effects of functional impairments. More importantly, social support did not have an impact on the pain–depression relationship. The moderator or the buffer model of social support received very qualified validation in this study. In an earlier study involving 875 chronic disease patients, specific types of social support did not add significantly to the prediction of better mental health outcomes over and above the effect of generic social support (Sherbourne and Hays, 1990)

In the final study in this section, Cronan and associates (1998) sought to determine whether experimentally developed social support, instruction in appropriate use of the health care system, or both were effective in reducing health care costs for 363 subjects with osteoarthritis (the only study not involving RA subjects reported here). They were randomly assigned to one of three intervention groups. Heath status and health care utilization were assessed at the point of entry after one, two, and three years. Health care costs in the combined experimental group were lower than those in the control group. The three interventions had nearly equal effects on health status and health care costs.

In short, social support alone was no more or no less effective than other kinds of intervention, except in one respect. When social support was combined with education, the group had less attrition and greater persistence. This was an experimental design with very hard measures of outcome. Social support alone was not as effective as when it was combined with other types of interventions.

Summary

We have avoided a critical review of the research literature primarily because this volume is aimed at a clinical readership and because excellent reviews are available for that purpose (deRiddler and Schreurs, 1996; Penninx *et al.*, 1996). On the other hand, despite some data to the contrary, which we have reported, we have drawn the correct conclusion that social support, on the whole, is beneficial and the support-buffer paradigm is now generally viewed as valid. The protective or the buffering function of social support in mitigating depression in patients with RA, on the basis of this review, appears to have considerable validity. A few points are worthy of reiteration. Although it is not always explicitly stated, the fact is that the support provider is, more often than not, in an intimate relationship with the patient. In general, this individual is either the spouse or the partner. Research studies do not always identify specifically the identity of support providers. Social support has to be distinguished from network support, although both types have their value. From a clinical point of view, these studies make a strong case for social intervention to shore up the support system or at least to examine the nature of the support system available to the patient.

A handful of studies have raised doubts about the general acceptance of the stress-buffer role of social support. Social support has been shown to be an overarching concept that needs to be broken down to specific types of support. Spousal support, commonly regarded as the most readily available as well as a more effective type of social support, is shown to be less than desirable, but not in terms of spousal reinforcement of illness behaviors, which has been the focus in the pain literature.

Another point is that in relation to RA patients, social support research shows a preoccupation with the power of social support to eliminate or reduce the level of depression, to the exclusion of overall functioning of the patient, or with the power of social support to moderate illness behaviors. This is clearly a gap in the literature. It is reasonable to assume that if a patient is in a supportive environment and not subject to depression he or she will function more effectively. Research rarely takes that extra step to show the benefits that may accrue from social support in the larger arena of patient, as well as family, functioning.

SOCIAL SUPPORT AND HEADACHE

The literature on the role of social support and headache is a collection of studies without the benefit of a central theme, such as testing the buffering role of social support. The literature is more concerned with lack of social support or the need for its availability. Martin and Theunissen (1993) compared 28 subjects with chronic headaches with two individually matched control groups in terms of life-events, stress, coping skills, and social support. The headache group scored significantly lower on social support compared to the control groups. No differences were found on life-events stress or coping between the groups. The authors suggested that clinicians should make some effort to mobilize social support, and that effective social support should be considered a desirable treatment goal.

Lack or ineffective use of social support was noted in a study of 87 undergraduates with recurrent tension headaches compared to 177 in a matched control group (Holm et al., 1986). Headache subjects relied on ineffective coping strategies of avoidance and self-blame, and made less use of social support than did the normal controls. In another study involving Australian and American undergraduate students, a major finding was that the prevalence of headache was three to four times higher among American students than their Australian counterparts (Martin and Nathan, 1987). A greater incidence of stressors and a deficient social support system accounted for much of the difference between the two groups.

It is not just the ineffective use of social support that is problematic, but a lack of satisfaction with the available support was the finding of a study involving 62 adult chronic headache sufferers and 64 nonheadache controls (Martin and Soon, 1993). However, support measures did not reveal any linear relationship with headache chronicity. They made a plea for greater attention from clinicians and researchers to the social dimension of headache. Another study noted poorer social support in 24 female patients with cluster headache compared to randomly selected and age-matched migraine sufferers (Blomkvist *et al.*, 1997). However, cluster headache patients were found to be significantly more positive as to their anticipated activities in the future compared to the migraine patients. It is conceivable that other means of coping could minimize or even eliminate the need for effective social support.

The quality of the studies relating headache and social support is quite different from the group of studies with RA. The consequences or lack of ineffective social support are not addressed. These studies on the whole failed to make a compelling case for the value of social support, and relied on the proposition of the intrinsic merit of such support. Nevertheless, a couple of these studies make a strong plea that social dimensions of headaches, including social support, should be an integral part of a clinical investigation.

LOW-BACK PAIN AND SOCIAL SUPPORT

A handful of studies investigated the influence of social support on CLBP. These studies generally confirmed the value of social support in coping with CLBP. Social support appears to have the capacity to enable CLBP patients to gain good pain control. That was one of the findings of a study involving 95 African–American CLBP patients (Klapow *et al.*, 1995). Twenty-five subjects categorized with chronic pain syndrome reported greater life adversity, more reliance on passive–avoidant coping strategies, and a less satisfactory network. In contrast, subjects reporting good pain control reported less adversity, less reliance on passive–avoidant coping strategies, and more satisfactory social support network. A third group comprising 24 subjects presented a mixed picture to the extent that they reported less life adversity, but more reliance on passive–avoidant coping strategies and more satisfactory social support network. Their adaptation to pain was positive. Two points are noteworthy. First, a social support network was only one of the psychosocial factors predicting good pain control; second, the concept of social support network has to be distinguished from intimate social support alluded to throughout this chapter.

A Swedish study that looked beyond intimate social support and involved a nonclinical population of 90 registered nurses found that social support from coworkers, in addition to psychological demands, authority over decisions, and skill utilization, had a significant effect on symptoms of low-back pain (Ahlberg-Hulten and Theorell, 1995). However, neck and shoulder pain were related to support at work only. The latter finding was telling in terms of the role of social support in mitigating shoulder and neck pain. However, from a theoretical or clinical perspective, the reasons for social support being more effective with one kind of pain than another are not clear.

In another Swedish study, involving 22,180 employees, 31% reported neck pain and 39% reported back pain. Lifting, monotonous work tasks, vibration, and uncomfortable work postures were the most important ergonomic factors. Work content and social support were the critical psychosocial factors. The combination of poor psychosocial work environment and exposure to one of the ergonomic variables produced the highest risk factors. In other words, inadequate social support emerged as a very critical factor in predicting high risk for back pain.

Trief and colleagues (1995) investigated the role of social support in the mitigation of depression in 70 patients with CLBP. The depressed patients differed from the nondepressed patients in their perceived social support and family environment. A noteworthy finding was that depression did not appear to have any association with rehabilitation outcomes. Clearly, susceptibility to depression in CLBP patients is related to the availability of social support, and to that extent this study furnishes further evidence for the stress-buffer model for social support.

It is virtually impossible to draw any general conclusions on the basis of a handful of rather varied studies on social support and CLBP. While these studies confirm the usefulness of social support in preventing depression or coping more effectively with pain, they are extraordinarily varied in scope and methodology. From a clinical perspective, they lend further credence to the necessity of careful assessment of the patient's social support system. We shall shift our focus to the issue of clinical application and usefulness of social support in our work with chronic pain sufferers.

CLINICAL ISSUES

The loss of a support system for chronic pain patients, especially those seen in pain clinics, is sadly a common tale. Common sense dictates that persistent and severe pain narrows or eliminates social interaction. When job loss is added, the sense of isolation for some patients becomes almost as intolerable as the pain itself.

As a starting point, we briefly address the nature of interaction between an individual and the social support system. It is convenient to visualize the support system as informal, semiformal, and formal. Within the confines of the informal system, it is usual to have partners, close relatives, children, parents, grandparents, and perhaps close friends. The semiformal system is represented by work, church, stores, voluntary organizations, family physicians, and so on. The formal system consists of medical services, workers compensation boards, unemployment insurance, Canada Pension, courts, police, and so on. Close listening to the patient reveals an interesting pattern in relation to the social system network. The informal and semiformal systems shrink, and interaction with the formal systems increases. The support literature has correctly emphasized the spouse as the most important source of support. However, not infrequently we encounter patients who are single through divorce, widowhood, or choice.

Singleness and Social Support: The situation of a single person and social support is well illustrated by a 56-year-old divorced woman who came to our clinic with unremitting neck and shoulder pain. She was unemployed, but was engaged in a mortal combat with her former employer of 26 years. She was convinced that her pain problems were work related, but, of course, her employers were not, and so she became enmeshed in the web of medical investigations required by her former employer. In addition, she is trying to obtain a disability pension, since she has no way to support herself. Although she can ill afford one, the lady has retained a lawyer. The woman does have a married son and one grandson.

Before suffering her pain conditions, she had a busy and fulfilling life. Her work to her was much more than a living, it was at the very center of her social life. Loss of employment meant loss of her social life and many friends. She explained that in the early stages of her illness, friends from work used to call her to join them in going out to shows and restaurants. Pain usually prevented her from joining them; after a while invitations stopped. She visits her son and daughter-in-law on weekends and does have a close relationship with them. But, they are quite busy and could not fill the void left by the loss of job and workmates. We are encouraging her to join the local Chronic Pain Society and other support organizations in her community, but she has shown little enthusiasm for these activities. This case is important because with such strong importance attached to intimate relationships in the support literature, the role that friends and work tend to play in the absence of a spouse as means of support is often overlooked.

This Is Not What I Expected: We next relate the story of a single businesswoman who sold her lucrative business at age 65 to spend more time with her mother and to pursue her lifelong dream of travel with her sister. Within a year of selling her business, her mother died, and soon after that the woman developed severe backache, for which she was extensively investigated but with no definitive findings. When she came to our clinic, she was living as a virtual recluse.

Her pain had completely taken over her life, and she spent all her time within her house. She was not eating well, and there was evidence of depression.

Over time she revealed that the sudden death of her mother had turned her life upside down. When she developed severe back pain, she almost lost her will to live. She disconnected from all her social activities and refused to see her sister. With her mother's death her support system simply evaporated. One might speculate about the onset of her back pain so soon after her mother's death. Grief and pain often go hand in hand, but her isolation, largely self-imposed, was significant. She was placed on antidepressant medication, and a major effort was made to reconnect her with significant persons in her life. A teenage volunteer helped her shop and run errands. Her sister became involved, and she gradually reconnected with some of her lifelong friends from the business world. Her mood and her pain improved and she was discharged from the pain clinic. At that time she was planning a trip abroad with her sister.

The unexpected death of an intimate, pain, depression, and the ensuing isolation basically summarize this case. With little actual medical intervention but considerable psychiatric and psychosocial, input, this woman was restored to her premorbid level of functioning. Restoration of her social network and support was a central feature of the treatment.

A CASE OF SOLID SOCIAL SUPPORT

Is She Sick or Not? Another familiar phenomenon observed at pain clinics is uncertainty about the diagnosis, which only complicates the nature of support, already frequently characterized by ambivalence. We relate the case of a husband and wife engaged in couple therapy. The patient is a 42-year-old woman diagnosed with fibromyalgia. Based on his reading of the subject and conversations with physicians, her husband has many questions about the medical value of this diagnosis He has undergone inner conflicts about his wife's level of disability, and he vacillates from sympathy and support to doubting the source, and even validity, of her pain. His wife said that his attitude varies with the weather, or the kind of day he had at work, or if their children are playing up. The situation was further complicated by the almost daily change in the patient's feelings and activity level. Hence, consistent emotional and practical support by her husband was practically impossible. His attitude brought them into therapy.

Can Social Support Be Any Better? A young woman was diagnosed with RA which rapidly progressed and she had to leave her job as a veterinarian's assistant. She was referred to the pain clinic by her family physician because she was going through a difficult time coming to terms with her altered circumstances. She came from a well-to-do family, being the younger of two siblings. Her lifelong dream was to work with horses. She could not remember a time when she did not ride horses.

The woman had been married only a short time at the time of her diagnosis. She and her husband were seen together to evaluate his attitude to her condition and the fact that her condition deteriorated so rapidly. Only in his twenties, he was remarkably composed and matter of fact. He announced that he loved his wife and would have married her anyway. He was very optimistic that her condition would improve, and she would find many ways of leading a fulfilled life. He was there for her.

Soon after, he gave up his job and started his own business. This move proved to be highly positive for the patient. She ran the office from home. She decided to take a computer course to learn basic accounting. Through all of this her parents, to whom our patient was very close, gave her an enormous amount of emotional and practical support. Her father became involved in helping her husband get the business properly set up. Her older brother, who lived 800 miles away, telephoned her frequently and visited her often.

In the arena of formal support, she remained in supportive psychotherapy at the pain clinic for about a year. Her family physician as well as her rheumatologist made significant contributions to help her deal with her illness. Fortunately, she responded well to an experimental drug, and her pain and functioning showed signs of improvement.

A supportive husband combined with a highly caring family and health care professionals created an optimal environment for support. It is difficult to judge how rare is this level of support. Also noteworthy is this patient's determination to carry on. Psychotherapy helped her to change directions and goals, which she found to be the most difficult challenge.

Widowhood and Loss of Support: A 56-year-old woman was referred to the pain clinic for unremitting tension headaches which remained impervious to medical intervention and apparently disabling her. Questioning this patient revealed the dramatic and totally unexpected death of her husband. He rang the doorbell one evening, and by the time our patient answered the door he was slumped over and died soon after from a massive coronary infarction. This event took place two years before her inception at our clinic. She had been a homemaker all her life, raising a son and a daughter. Her husband, an excellent provider, was also very much the decision maker, and his wife relied heavily on him.

His death left her without the only significant support in her life. To make matters worse, her son got involved in minor criminal activities, was caught, and put on probation. Her daughter was in a state of doldrums, having dropped out of school, apparently without any future plans. It was during this time that the patient's headaches deteriorated. Apart from psychotherapy and group therapy for pain management, a key element of the treatment was to help her to reintegrate into the community. Her entire social life revolved around her husband's. She did not have any close friends. In time, this woman made a remarkable recovery. She discovered many hidden talents, took complete charge of her family finances, made one or two close friends from the therapy group, told her children that they had to straighten up or they could expect no ongoing help from her. Her headaches subsided to the point that she was free of medication.

This patient story is instructive because her entire active involvement with the health care system was triggered by the tragic loss of her husband, her only source of support. She had relied almost entirely on him for emotional and every other kind of support. She informed the therapist that she had never paid a bill, never handled family finances, or made decisions about anything important. She was quite happy to leave such matters to her husband. With the help of the pain clinic, which became her main source of support for the next two years, she developed into a self-reliant and confident individual, making friends and discovering her own hidden strengths.

SUMMARY

Social support plays a buffering role in moderating depression in RA. The headache and CLBP literature lacks the direction in research evident in the RA literature. Perhaps social and chronic pain research has been distracted by the debate over the role of the spouse in the reinforcement of pain behavior. The buffering role of social support against depression or pain in the chronic pain patient has received limited support. The consequences for lack of support were investigated in a few studies. There was general acknowledgment that from a clinical perspective social support was an important dimension that ought to be investigated.

The case illustrations highlighted that point. It is undeniable that chronic illness alters the nature of social interaction. Informal and semiformal may shrink, while the interaction with the formal network is on the rise (see Table 7.1). Spouses and family members are required to assume a significant level of responsibility as the patient becomes more and more dependent on them. On the other hand, when spouses and family members are simply unavailable, then the support system for the patient must be found elsewhere. Work for many of these patients is much more than a living. We have observed over many years that unemployment due to pain and disability for these individuals has serious consequences. Mobilization of social support for some of the patients described here was just as critical in their overall treatment for pain as was medication and physiotherapy or any other intervention. These patients found themselves alone with pain and, not infrequently, a hostile world in the health care system, past employers, and institutions that provide financial assistance. Social isolation and grief leading to pain symptoms brought some of these patients to our clinic.

Unraveling those facts and acting on them yielded positive results. Yet the evidence is only anecdotal in relation to chronic pain patients. Some satisfaction can be drawn from the observation that outside of the chronic pain literature, the buffering role of social support is reasonably well established. Clinicians working with chronic pain patients need not be unduly discouraged by the lack of significant empirical support for the merit of social support in the chronic pain literature.

Chapter 8

CHRONIC PAIN PATIENT AND THE OCCUPATIONAL ROLE

INTRODUCTION

The value of work is undeniable. Work is not only a means to an end, but not infrequently it is an end in itself. We live in a society where the Protestant work ethic has very deep roots. Many pejorative terms exist to describe individuals who do not conform to this fundamental requirement of gainful employment. In recent times, unemployment has come to be viewed not as an economic fallout of ebbs and flows of the capitalist system but as personal failure. This is evident in legislative changes in Canada, for example, where, as a first step, unemployment insurance was renamed employment insurance, and resultant changes in the legislation deprived thousands of unemployed persons of this entitlement. Britain is making similar changes. Welfare is now workfare. In this climate, the inability to work due to obscure chronic pain problems confronts our patients with untold misery and shame, as evident in the cases of Mrs. Abrams (Chapter 1) and Mr. Bloom (Chapter 2). First, there is the shame of losing a highly valued role, and, second, the failure to convince the powers that be that inability to work is based on legitimate medical problems.

In Chapter 2 we reviewed the economic cost of unemployment along with the depression related to unemployment. In this chapter we broaden the scope and first examine the concept of occupational role, which in some ways transcends merely paid employment, followed by the broad issue of job loss due to disability, and return to work as a measure of success in the treatment of chronic pain patients. A recent report on back pain in the workplace raised some controversial issues of disability due to chronic back pain and the need for reconceptualization of the very notion of what may constitute pain (Fordyce, 1995). Disability arising out of chronic low-back pain of uncertain origin may not be attributable to pain but to psychological causes. We shall return to this report in subsequent chapters. We provide case illustrations to highlight clinical issues that arise when the occupational roles of our patients are threatened or lost.

This chapter and the next two share a common theme, namely the reasons for losing paid employment due to chronic pain conditions. Physicians are often at the heart of the issue, since it is their judgment that determines the eligibility. Workers compensation boards and insurance companies rely almost entirely on medical opinion for their final disposition. However, we emphasize somewhat different issues in all three chapters, but the binding theme remains the inability of the worker to function due to chronic pain.

THE COMPLEXITIES OF THE SICK ROLE AND THE OCCUPATIONAL ROLE

We consider some common problems reported by our patients concerning occupational roles. Women face some unique problems in society. The vast majority of women are in the workforce, and most of them continue to carry a substantial portion of homemaking activities. Job loss for them, especially single parents, has enormous implications. We shall attempt to draw out some of the specifics in relation to occupational role as reported by our patients and supported by the literature.

First, we revisit the concept of sick role, and the specifics of occupational role through a selected review of the literature. The concept of sick role is inextricably intertwined with occupational role. Sick role has four elements. Two of these are in the category of rights, and two in the category of obligations. First, and this has serious implication for pain patients, the sick individual is not responsible for being ill and is certainly not to be blamed for the condition. This presents a special problem for our patients because the legitimacy of their conditions is often questioned. The aforementioned report on back pain even concluded that most chronic back pain sufferers are victims of psychological or emotional distress. While the report emphasized the rarity of malingering, many of our patients are left with the impression that their pain complaints are not legitimate. Hence, inability to work is often viewed with suspicion by all parties. Our patient is now confronted with a major loss, and that suffering is compounded by the questionable nature of the medical complaint: Is the person ill? The first element of the sick role is thus challenged for many chronic pain patients.

The second element is the right of the patient to be exempted from her or his usual obligations, whatever they may be. This is problematic, especially so for female patients, whose obligations as mother, spouse, and homemaker may not be quite so easily suspended without serious repercussions. Overwhelming evidence exists from Africa to the United States that women, in or out of the workforce, perform most of the domestic work (gender-based occupational role) (Charles and Hopflinger, 1992; Marcoux, 1994). There is further evidence that role-related stressors are significantly enhanced for working mothers in their effort to combine occupational and parental roles (Luchetta, 1995). Thomas (1997) observed that in their effort to enact the roles of mothers, wives, and workers, many women succumb to physical and mental distress. Some women allegedly choose the sick role as a means to escape from the demands of their multiple roles. For patients with young children exemption from these duties is practically impossible. The point is that women cannot altogether escape from their role obligations even in the face of poor health as envisaged by the sick role.

As our case illustration shows, for a female chronic pain patient failure to perform domestic and child-rearing functions has serious fallouts. For those in full-time paid employment, leave from work is only the first step, which not infrequently culminates in termination. Failure or serious impairment in the occupational role has been demonstrated to have far-reaching negative effects on marriage in a mentally ill population (Claussen, 1981). This study found a strong association between job loss and dissolution of marriage. A short-term right often becomes a long-term conflict within families, and almost always with the external world. This process involves transition from the sick role to the chronic sick role. We shall presently discuss the ramifications of the latter.

The third element is an obligation associated with the sick role, and the obligation is for the patient to behave in a manner that suggests that being ill is unacceptable and undesirable. Social expectation is for this individual to recover and return to normal functioning. In relation to this obligation, our patients face a challenging problem. Most seem to act and behave in the socially desirable direction and want to be rid of the affliction and return to normal activities. Many succeed in the short run. The story is quite different in the long run.

The fourth and final element is another obligation for the patient to seek appropriate help. Common sense dictates that our patients seek medical help, but often it does not restore health. The failure to recover is filled with peril for our patients, and they often receive much disaffection and even the wrath of the medical profession, family, and other institutions.

The chronic sick role modifies some duties and obligations of the sick role. Gallagher and Wrobel (1982) observed that "unlike acute problems such as most infectious diseases or broken bones, chronic diseases are long term and ongoing, often with little likelihood of cure." This is certainly true of most patients with chronic pain conditions. In addition, the diagnostic uncertainty with our patients, unlike chronic collagen or cardiovascular disorders, is a source of stress. In other words, our patients must prove their disabilities.

Gallagher (1976) advanced the idea that in chronic conditions which lead to chronic sick role, adaptation rather than cure is the most favorable outcome for the patient. This extension of the original sick role modifies societal expectation of the occupants of chronic sick role. On the other hand, for many patients with chronic pain, the legitimacy of their chronic sick role is readily questioned. This dilemma is evident in the IASP report on back pain in the workplace, where they assert that "the concept of disability has broadened (in relation to chronic back pain) to include matters difficult to assess and that have gone well beyond the original intent of what constitutes a compensable disability" (Fordyce, 1995). Implicit in that statement is that difficult matters to assess somehow become suspect and the question of whether they are able to work, is regularly asked of chronic pain sufferers. From the patient's point of view the loss of the occupational role, which is in itself a painful experience, is compounded by doubts about the legitimacy of their pain by the patient, family, friends, and medical profession.

A CASE SURROUNDED BY DOUBTS

Mrs. Hanson, age 40, was the victim of an automobile accident in which she sustained back and head injuries. Extensive neurological and orthopedic investigations failed to establish any lasting damage from the injuries. However, she developed severe migraine-type headaches and mild back pain. Mrs. Hanson had been a busy mother, spouse, full-time legal secretary, and engaged in several voluntary activities. She was free of any health problems. The accident changed all that. She became housebound and, in her own words, a prisoner of her pain. When first seen at the pain clinic, she seemed filled with grief over the partial loss of parental and spousal activities and a total loss of her occupational role. She displayed an extraordinary amount of guilt over her disability. A year and a half after the accident she managed to obtain part-time employment, but was terrified of losing it. Her fear was based in reality, because her headaches, which were not infrequent, rendered her incapable of any activities.

Her family consisted of her husband, a professional engineer, 14-year-old son John, and 10-year-old daughter Sue. Her husband's job required some travel. Mr. Hanson depended on his wife for all family responsibilities, from taking care of family finances to maintaining contact with the children's school. He was devastated by her accident and mystified by the degree of her disability. It was the uncertain nature of the headaches that caused such confusion. One day she could function almost at a normal level, but the very next day she would have difficulty just getting out of bed. This situation caused much distress in the family, but the main victim was Mrs. Hanson.

For women, work and domestic responsibilities are sources of stress, but the loss of those roles completely or in part, is even more stressful. For Mrs. Hanson, managing her family affairs was sometimes hard, but her inability to work for such a long time after the accident did not give her a sense of relief (secondary gain, discussed in Chapter 9) but significantly added to her distress: in fact, she became depressed. She had enjoyed her work and had a close working relationship with her lawyer employers. Some evidence exists that the nature of the secretary–employer relationship determines the level of satisfaction (Harvey, 1976).

Although unable to work, Mrs. Hanson could not cease being a homemaker and mother. These roles created a great deal of tension between she and her husband, and to a lesser extent with the children. Conceptually, much of the confusion arose directly out of the legitimacy of Mrs. Hanson's sick role. Finerman and Bennett (1995) analyzed the shift in Western medicine to placing responsibility and blame for disease on the victims. This problem is multiplied several-fold when the nature of the disease itself is suspect. This redefinition also poses a direct challenge to the Parsonian notion of sick role, which has so far stood the test of time. For the patient the situation can become truly untenable. Mrs. Hanson, apart from coping with multiple losses, now had to justify her disability, mostly to herself. Against this background, it is perhaps less than surprising that she harbored an inordinate amount of guilt and succumbed to depression.

A most significant issue not always explicit in research literature is that loss of the occupational role has different implications for women and men, and that this loss is often one of several. We now briefly review the specifics of Mrs. Hanson's case in relation to her pain condition and the losses that ensued. Mrs. Hanson did not work for a year and a half following her accident. Mr. Hanson and, to a lesser extent, John were greatly mystified by the level of her disability. Initially, Mr. Hanson's reaction to her inability to work was positive. Financially, they were reasonably well off and not dependent on Mrs. Hanson's wages. Mr. Hanson's unexpressed (he only revealed it during conjoint therapy) expectation was that she would have more time for the children and her community activities. In other words, he regarded her job loss almost as a voluntary act which would be beneficial. His denial of her pain and distress was almost total. He failed to see his wife's profound sense of loss at losing her job.

Of course, the problem was further complicated when, contrary to his expectation, she was less than effective at running their household. This was the beginning of their marital conflict, which eventually brought them to this writer's office. It did not take long for Mr. Hanson to realize that his wife's termination of employment did not make her more available to the rest of the family, but her whole behavior became unpredictable. She was far less reliable than she had ever been in their marriage, and he was having to do more. Besides, he couldn't be sure of the state in which he might find her when he returned from business trips. She might be confined to bed or up and about. This uncertainty led the children to refrain from inviting their friends home, lest the noise made her headaches worse, and it caused her husband much dismay and anger. From Mr. Hanson's perspective, she was not pulling her weight, and he was still unwilling to give her the benefit of doubt as far as her headaches were concerned.

This case illustrates some of the more common problems encountered by female sufferers of benign chronic pain conditions of uncertain origin. Loss of her occupational role was virtually explained away by Mr. Hanson, but when her domestic responsibilities began to suffer he became angry and questioned the legitimacy of her pain and disability. Concerning the sick role and the obligations and privileges associated with it, Mrs. Hanson failed in one critical dimension. She did not meet the expectation that she would recover and resume normal functioning. As for her right to occupy the chronic sick role, there was total lack of consensus among the medical profession, which in turn significantly colored the view of Mr. Hanson. The net effect was that Mrs. Hanson became totally demoralized and culminated in her psychological decompensation.

We now explore the case of a male chronic pain sufferer to determine the impact of the loss of the occupational role, and we note the distinction from Mrs. Hanson's case. Mr. Hinkley, 58 years old, was involved in a workplace accident that injured his back. He was given paid medical leave, and after about a month he returned to work. Soon after, his pain returned, and he was forced to apply for disability benefits, which were denied. He had the usual medical investigations, which failed to establish any lasting damage to his back from the accident. He was forced to take early retirement.

He reacted to his job loss by an inordinate amount of anger, which was mainly vented at his wife. There children were grown and had limited contact with their parents. Mr. Hinkley had led a restricted life, and the forced retirement had some negative consequences for him. His marriage was a traditional one. Mrs. Hinkley had never worked outside the house. Mr. Hinkley now began to neglect his areas of responsibility (managing the money, doing outside work, and helping his wife). Mrs. Hinkley complained that he had had a personality change. She was afraid to say anything to him, lest he should lose his temper. She quietly took over his chores, and he not so quietly progressed toward chronicity and disability. When seen at the pain clinic, he refused to participate in the rehabilitation program on the grounds that what he needed was relief from his back pain and not some "fancy" program.

This is broadly the gist of the case. His early retirement caused some financial difficulties, but it was his change in demeanor that caused his wife much distress. He was able to slip into the chronic sick role without much resistance from any source. One tenet of the chronic sick role is that the patient should be enabled to perform at his or her optimal level. Mr. Hinkley, by his refusal to engage in rehabilitation, denied himself that opportunity. His anger at "unjust" treatment by his employer and the medical profession, which robbed him of one of his most meaningful roles, was so overwhelming that he refused any further involvement with the health care system. She also assumed some of his family-related duties.

Unlike Mrs. Hanson, Mr. Hinkley's loss of occupational role was far less disruptive to the family system. The Hinkleys' age also contributed to the changes in the family organization. Mrs. Hinkley's willingness to take over her husband's part of the domestic arrangement (which were quite nominal) allowed smooth, though perhaps not desirable, transition. The major change occurred in the affective involvement between the couple.

From being a relatively engaged husband, he became aloof. The efficiency with which this family ran before his trauma basically remained unchanged. This case was selected to lend credence to the argument that chronic illness in a male is likely to be somewhat less disruptive than in a female. However, it should be recognized that job loss in men can, and often does, have far-reaching consequences, as illustrated by Mr. Bloom in Chapter 2. This man's job loss created huge family problems and he eventually committed suicide. Yet, the overwhelming evidence is that for women faced with chronic illness, it is that much harder to relinquish homemaking and child-rearing activities than for men. A key point is that so much of a person's identity is tied up with the job that when job loss occurs due to a chronic pain condition, the person faces the illegitimacy of the medical condition and loss of an extraordinary valuable role. Most patients report a great sense of humiliation combined with profound sadness.

TREATMENT OUTCOME AND THE OCCUPATIONAL ROLE

A common measure in the outcome literature on chronic pain is the restoration of the occupational role. Other measures include reduction in medication, uptime hours, and, most important, pain relief through medication and psychological techniques. In this section we concentrate on return to work as the outcome measure. We also explore the merit of this variable as a measure of treatment success.

It is hard to dispute that restoration of the occupational role is highly desirable. However, common sense dictates that return to work could be a harsh measure of success for many patients given the intractable and elusive nature of chronic pain. Other than the objective of return to work, these studies are extraordinarily varied methodology and treatment programs.

Multidisciplinary treatment programs for chronic pain have goals that mostly go beyond just return to work, but include measures such as improvements in pain, mood, activity level, reduction in medication intake, uptime hours, and so on. Nevertheless, several such treatment programs have reported return to work directly attributable to their treatment. Flor *et al.*, (1992) conducted a meta analysis of 65 studies to evaluate the effectiveness of multidisciplinary pain treatment. A detailed analysis of the behavioral class of outcome variables revealed that there were substantial effects of the treatments on measures such as return to work and utilization of the health care system. Concerning return to work, treated patients had a 68% probability to return to work compared with 32% for the untreated. This important review clearly established that those treated at the multidisciplinary pain clinics were likely to make significantly more gains than patients who did not. An earlier analysis of the literature on coping with chronic pain (Jensen *et al.*, 1991) reported that patients who believed that they were able to control their pain, who avoided catastrophizing, and who believed that they were not severely disabled appeared to function better than those who did not. In other words, the patients' belief system combined with personality factors were the most telling determinants of positive outcome. In the final analysis, the patient was the author of his or her own fortune or misfortune.

Deardorff and coworkers (1991) compared 42 chronic pain patients treated at a multidisciplinary pain management program with 15 patients who did not participate. Comparisons were made at the point of entry and at a follow-up 11 months later. Twenty-five of the treated patients and seven of the untreated patients had return to work as their goal. Twelve (48%) of the 25 patients returned to work, and an additional 7 (28%) patients were involved in vocational rehabilitation or were being interviewed for jobs. None of the untreated group with return to work as a goal achieved their objective. The authors emphasized that return to work was a stringent criterion measure because it encompassed many higher levels of functional ability beyond those assessed at discharge. Another point was the emphasis on the patient's motivation to return to work. At the time of this study the return-to-work results ranged from 15% to 100%, with an average of 55% returning to work or vocational rehabilitation (Deardorff *et al.*, 1991).

A more recent study reported on 90 patients with chronic low-back pain who participated in a multidisciplinary pain management program (Pfingsten *et al.*, 1997). The main therapeutic goal of this program was to facilitate return to work. All subjects were measured at the beginning and end of the program. First and foremost, the combined functional and psychological treatment resulted in significant improvements among most patients by the end of the program. Interestingly, self-evaluation of return to work was the most powerful indicator for returning to work. Return to work did not materialize in 70% of cases in which patients believed before treatment that return to work was not feasible. One plausible conclusion is that the treatment program was not altogether successful in remotivating patients to return to work.

Another study investigated motivation of returning to work in a group of 168 patients with chronic low-back pain (Carosella *et al.*, 1994). Subjects were divided as follows: those who completed the 4-week, 5-day-per-week program ($n = 84$) and those who were discharged before completing the program ($n = 84$). Subjects who completed the program demonstrated a higher expectation to return to work, and less disability, somatization, and pain intensity than did the treatment dropout group. Note, however, that this was a work-hardening program with strict time limits and expectations. The authors emphasized the importance of the expectations for reentry into the workforce in an intervention targeted at rehabilitation and return to work.

Tan and associates (1997) also found that the goal of return to work was the single best predictor for return-to-work outcome in a group of subjects with chronic musculoskeletal pain. Age, education, and marital status were also predictive for return-to-work outcome. However, the most powerful predictor was the motivation for returning to work. Dozios and associates (1995) examined which variables may predict return to work in 117 patients with work-related low-back pain. Psychological factors, such as pain and disability perception, coping strategies, and depression at the time of admission, were the most critical variables that predicted return to work. Physical status and the subject's perception of disability predicted return to work following treatment. In short, those who viewed themselves as not disabled by pain were able to return to work.

The success of work hardening to return patients with chronic low-back pain to work was also reported in a brief paper by Ricke *et al.*, (1995). A total of 32 patients received this treatment; at the two-month follow-up, 21 subjects returned to their old jobs, 6 worked at different jobs, and 5 were unable to return to work. The effectiveness of this program was highlighted.

Sanders and Brena (1993) administered Sickness Impact Profile, Medical Examination and Diagnostic Information Coding System, and treatment outcome measures to 180 chronic pain patients. All patients participated in a multidisciplinary pain rehabilitation program. The results of multidimensional cluster analyses identified four subgroups:

1. Cluster A: highly dysfunctional with moderate level of physical pathology;
2. Cluster B: moderately dysfunctional with moderate levels of physical pathology;
3. Cluster C: highly functional with low levels of physical pathology;
4. Cluster D: highly dysfunctional with low levels of physical pathology.

Clusters A and D patients showed the most improvement in several areas, including paid work at follow-up. Cluster C patients were the next best, showing improvements in all areas except activity level. Cluster B patients showed the least improvement. The authors noted that their findings agreed with previous research that found differential effectiveness of treatment as a function of subgroup. Their conclusion was that the study offered real support for the application of clustering methods, and this was especially useful in relation to return to work for chronic pain patients.

Gatchel *et al.* (1995) reported on 324 patients with acute low-back pain and their propensity for chronicity. A follow-up interview at six months after the psychological assessment evaluated return-to-work status. The factors that differentiated patients who were back at work versus those who were not revealed that self-reported disability, a personality disorder, and some specific findings on the Minnesota Multiple Personality Inventory were predictive of those who failed to return and fell into the chronicity trap. Their conclusion was that the presence of specific psychosocial factors in injured workers was predictive of chronicity. This study makes an important contribution by emphasizing the self-reported aspect of disability. Psychological and personality factors distinguished those with a propensity for chronicity from those who returned to normal living.

SUMMARY

There is no way to exaggerate the importance of work in a modern society. No other single role has such profound impact on the individual than the loss of the occupational role. Even when parental or spousal roles are compromised, they do not carry the societal sanctions that job loss does. This emphasis on work goes beyond the person's ability to support himself and his family, but it is viewed as a matter of great personal failure and abrogation of a social contract, and a certain amount of stigma is attached to not working. Hence, loss of this role has very serious psychological and social consequences for the individual and society.

When the loss of this role is perceived to be on illegitimate grounds, such as an elusive chronic pain condition, there are many societal sanctions. Being denied disability pay and being labeled a freeloader and irresponsible are examples of sanctions. Thus, our attitudes are shaped toward those who are not entirely up to the task. Societal attitude toward ill health has changed greatly since Parsons first articulated the concept of sick role. A most radical change in that conceptualization is the new emphasis on personal responsibility to maintain health. It is simply not enough to seek medical attention during illness. To what extent is an individual responsible for the illness? When illness is elusive, such as chronic pain syndrome, the patient is confronted with a two-edged sword: (1) the veracity of the condition itself; and (2) taking responsibility for the consequences of the condition (e.g., disability and job loss).

The latter is clearly evident in the preceding review. The two most critical factors that seem to mitigate against a chronic pain patient returning to work are (a) his or her motivation to return to work, and (b) psychological disturbance combined with certain personality characteristics. Motivation to return to work merits further scrutiny. The most glaring implication is that despite many factors (nature of disability, type of work, demographic factors), the determining factor is the desire of the patient to return to work. If for some reason that desire is diluted or doubts are expressed about one's ability to return to work, blame becomes a very real issue. Hence, many chronic pain patients are viewed as the authors of their misfortune and responsible for all the incidental problems that arise from unemployment.

When this fact is combined with the psychological and emotional state of these patients, we begin to appreciate the societal attitude toward them and their struggle. Acceptance of their medical condition itself becomes a matter of debate and doubt. The literature contains no discussion of those who failed to return to work. Once it is demonstrated that lack of motivation is the reason for their failure, perhaps any further discussion is fruitless. When lack of motivation is combined with the verdict of the Task Force on Back Pain in the Workplace (Fordyce, 1995)—that the major problem in nonspecific low-back pain (NSLBP) disability appears to be the medicalization of suffering—the fate of those who lose their jobs due to nonspecific pain conditions, is sealed.

Yet, there is a clear need to go beyond the narrow focus of these studies to search for other legitimate reasons that might explain the high rate of unemployment in the chronic pain population. The argument is this: a main objective of pain management clinics is to help patients return to work, to help those who cannot deal with guilt, attitudes of others, etc., and to adopt more positive approaches to maximize their functioning in every respect. Okifuji and associates (1998) observed that evaluation of return to work was extremely complex. Several factors (physical demands of the job, regional variation of the job market, availability of job accommodation, marketability of patients' skills, extent of wage replacement, and financial incentives) influenced the return-to-work outcome. The last two factors relate to a patient's motivation to return to work. Nevertheless, these authors pointed out that multidisciplinary pain clinic treatment produced significantly better results in returning patients to work than conventionally treated patients (Okifuji *et al.*, 1998).

Teasell and Finestone (1999) have raised some important issues about socioeconomic factors as they relate to work disability. They argued that, in addition to medical factors, socioeconomic factors related to the work status of an individual with chronic disease are age, education, occupation, and job status in the labor force. Work disability was not necessarily related to the severity of the symptoms of low-back pain, but rather to the demands of the workplace. Similarly, they observed that socioeconomic status tended to be associated with an increase in the frequency and severity of disability as well as the rate of progression to disability in patients with musculoskeletal disorders.

These key factors need to be incorporated in the overall treatment plan for chronic pain patients to broaden the base of variables that seem to affect outcome. Chronic pain may be quite tolerable in one kind of job situation and unbearable in another. This problem was manifested by a fireman who sustained a work-related injury and faced enormous opposition to reassignment due to the uncertain nature of the clinical findings. His employers were anxious for him to take early retirement, which he refused. Through active intervention of the pain clinic, his employers modified their view of his disability and agreed to reassign him. Obviously, given the degree of disability he experienced following the accident, he simply could not have functioned as a fireman, but there was nothing to prevent him from carrying out a desk job. This man did not lack motivation to continue working. He firmly believed that he could not do his old job, which required a high level of physical proficiency.

The absence of discernible and credible clinical findings is at the heart of some of the difficulties encountered by our patients. Psychological reasons are often invoked for their inability and unwillingness to work. These beliefs are reinforced by research findings and prestigious publications by highly credible organizations. This is despite the fact that not working has serious financial and social consequences for the patient and the family.

Chapter 9

DILEMMA OF INJURED PATIENTS: WHAT ENTITLES THEM TO COMPENSATION?

INTRODUCTION

Being in constant, sometimes severe, pain and struggling to prove the legitimacy of that pain to employers, workers compensation board (WCB), and insurance companies is a common experience for many of our patients. We begin with a case study. This case is typical of many chronic pain patients: a fully functioning human being suffers chronic pain (from a minor motor vehicle accident) which could not be accounted for by objective medical findings. We also consider the critical issue of whether financial settlement resolves chronic pain problems. In other words, if patients are motivated to exaggerate or even emulate pain conditions for financial gain, do they return to normal functioning once the settlements are achieved? This issue is intricately connected with the diagnostic problems associated with chronic benign pain. We discuss those issues in the next chapter. However, in the context of a patient's claim of financial benefits, which is at the center of employer–employee or worker–WCB conflict, we explore the complex issue of secondary gain. This psychological and, in the main, unconscious phenomenon is surrounded by much misunderstanding. At its simplest, secondary gain is often confused with emulation of illness for financial gain. This is a gross misinterpretation of a clinical tool of great value.

The controversy of secondary gain and malingering has a long history in the medical literature. Culpant and Taylor (1973) reported on a classification of 82 subjects referred by lawyers for psychiatric evaluation following accidental injury. About a third of the subjects were disabled by "neurotic" symptoms which were directly attributable to the accident. About half of the subjects were unconsciously motivated by the possibility of financial compensation and failed to improve or became worse until settlement of their claims. Only five subjects were frank malingerers. This paper remains contemporary in many ways. First, as our review shows, malingering is rare, and equally hard to identify. Second, psychological fallout of a trauma can be significant, although the term "neurotic" has fallen out of fashion. Third, unlike this study, settlements of financial claims do not seem to resolve pain or health problems.

MRS. INKSTER: AN UNSATISFACTORY CASE

Mrs. Inkster, a 53-year-old patient, was involved in an automobile accident three years before coming to the pain clinic, at which time she also stopped working. At the time of her accident she had been a senior office worker for a large corporation since the late seventies.

Mrs. Inkster came from a farming family and was the third of six children. Her father drank heavily on weekends and could become volatile and even violent. For the most part, however, he was a reasonable man and a good provider. Mrs. Inkster was a good student and desired to become a nurse. For reasons not altogether clear, she was unable to achieve her ambition and started working after she finished high school. She still maintained close contact with her mother and some of her siblings.

She married at 19 to a man with whom she enjoyed a close relationship. She separated from her husband only after the car accident. Her reasons for this separation were vague. She apparently decided to end her marriage when she realized that she could no longer remain sexually active; in fact she reported that she could not even "bear to be touched." Her husband was opposed to this separation, but she persuaded him finally to accept her decision. He never remarried, and though they live many hundreds of miles apart, they remain in touch. They have a son and two grandchildren, who also lived in Winnipeg. Her son was born prematurely and had serious medical problems during infancy. This time was difficult for our patient, and she took some time off work. She became depressed, but it is unclear if she was treated for it. There was another occasion when she sought psychiatric consultation for depression, but she was sufficiently well to continue to work.

She also had several surgeries over many years unrelated to her pain condition. In addition, she had two previous car accidents during the 1980s and one in 1997, following the accident that resulted in her disability.

Mrs. Inkster's pain condition was diagnosed by a rheumatologist as fibromyalgia. She was relieved to finally have a name for her condition, as she had begun to wonder if the pain was in her head. The diagnosis, however, did not resolve her fundamental problem of receiving disability benefits from her employers. They were not convinced that she could no longer work full-time. In the meantime, she had lost the main source of her social support. She was a very active member of her trade union and worked many hours a day helping fellow employees with their work-related and personal problems. All her friends were from her workplace, but over time they drifted away. She returned to Manitoba to be near her son. In the meantime her financial situation became increasingly precarious.

She was ordered by her employer to undergo a psychiatric assessment, the findings of which were inconclusive. The psychiatrist concluded that if malingering or partial malingering (exaggeration of symptoms) were not present, then Mrs. Inkster had both a psychiatric problem and a medical problem. For the psychiatric problem, he suggested that undifferentiated somatoform disorder was a possibility, which could be complicated by a mood disorder, since many chronic pain patients with pain disorder were subject to major depression. He went on to suggest that chronic pain could also be a variant of a depressive disorder, which was often masked.

The psychiatrist was unable to comment accurately on her actual abilities. He had observed during his interview that the patient was not distracted by her pain, and she gave no evidence of any impairment of attention, memory, and concentration. Furthermore, her capacity for enjoyment was unimpaired. He took note of her mobility as she walked with him from his office to another part of the hospital. In conclusion, he recommended that the patient be assessed by a rehabilitation medicine specialist for complete functional assessment. He found no significant psychiatric problem with Mrs. Inkster. Yet, he strongly suggested that the patient's claim of disability was not congruent with his observation of her behavior during the interview.

Summary

This case is a clear illustration of the dilemma that confronts our patients, their employers, and the insurance companies. Mrs. Inkster's pain and associated disability are undeniable. The etiology of fibromyalgia is unknown, and any claim of its origin as a consequence of a motor vehicle accident may be questionable. The disability associated with fibromyalgia is undeniable. Thomas and Roy (1999) have noted the difficulties these patients encounter in returning to work. Relatively few of these patients qualify for disability benefits. In general, insurance companies find such claims untenable. Psychiatric evaluation was deemed necessary because the medical diagnosis was unacceptable for ascertaining disability. Neither the diagnosis of fibromyalgia nor the psychiatric assessment, which contained some unfavorable comments from the patient's point of view of her functional capacity, provided convincing evidence to support her claim of long-term disability. Her behavior during her psychiatric assessment even raised the possibility of malingering or partial malingering. The only viable psychiatric diagnosis was somatoform disorder.

Having rejected fibromyalgia as a reason for granting long-term disability, her employer was now armed with possible psychiatric conditions, such as somatoform disorder or even malingering. The latter bordered on criminal behavior, and the former could not be justified as a compensable disorder. Medical investigation truly portrayed this patient in a questionable light, which only added to her distress and further convinced her that complaint and suffering were not taken seriously by her employer and the medical profession.

Diagnostic complexities associated with a nonmalignant chronic pain condition are at the center of our patient's conflict with employers and financial institutions. The message from the employer was straightforward: "You may have a problem, but it is not serious enough for us to grant you disability. Furthermore, we don't understand your behavior, because you do not always act as though you are in a great deal of pain. You are not depressed. Your physical problem is not that serious. Is it possible that you are not on the level?" The last question raises the issue of malingering.

Malingering is a rarity, as noted by the Commission on the Evaluation of Pain (1987). Furthermore, in an extensive review of this topic, Craig *et al.* (1998) observed that the challenge of identifying malingering is complicated by a whole host of factors, and that the base rate for this behavior is low. A paper written over 50 years ago revealed a different attitude (Schwartz, 1946). This author asserted that "simulation" (of illness following head injury) was much more common in cases in which litigation was a factor.

Unfortunately, that attitude, even in the face of data to the contrary, remains current. However, malingering remains rare. If she is not malingering, then could she have a mental illness, such as somatoform disorder, that truly could not be related to the accident? Mrs. Inkster's past history of depression suggests a predisposition to psychiatric morbidity. Perhaps, she is not just seeking financial gain, but also some emotional and other gains by maintaining her sick-role status. Note: financial "gain" is elusive since disability benefits never match the premorbid income. Loss of income is inevitable when patients receive disability benefits, which are secondary gains. In the next section, we review the literature on the effects of financial settlement on the health of chronic pain patients. We then discuss the pros and cons of secondary gains.

FINANCIAL COMPENSATION AND CHRONIC PATIENTHOOD

The important question is: "Is financial compensation sufficient motive for patients to embark on a path that leads to chronic pain and disability"? Lewy (1940), writing in the Bulletin of the Menninger Clinic, observed that "compensation neurosis" is created by the conviction of having been in a compensative accident. He asserted that "The problem is definitely less medicosomatic than psychological and sociological and compensation should be denied in every clear case of post-accident neurosis without permanent organic damage." Perhaps not so coincidentally, more that half a century later the IASP report on nonorganic back pain made a similar observation, asserting that such back conditions should not be viewed as medical problems but as sociological and psychological problems (Fordyce, 1995). However, we show that the relationship between trauma and compensation is more complex. As noted earlier, the seeming financial gain in the final analysis is truly a financial loss because disability benefits inevitably fall below the actual income of the patients. Mrs. Inkster, for example, has now joined the ranks of the poor. Failure to obtain disability only added to her mental anguish and made her overall health status worse.

In a well-known study Melzack and others (1985) compared 81 subjects with chronic pain conditions, of whom 27 were receiving compensation, with 64 subjects with musculoskeletal pain, 15 of whom were receiving compensation. On the Minnesota Multiple Personality Inventory (MMPI) and the McGill Pain Questionnaire (MPQ), the compensation and noncompensation groups obtained virtually identical scores. Compensation patients registered fewer visits to health professionals and scored lower on the affective dimension of the MPQ. This might have been an outcome of reduced anxiety and depression due to their more secure financial situation. The most important finding was that the patients on compensation were not psychologically distinguishable from noncompensation subjects. The authors made a strong case for treating patients awaiting litigation or on compensation with the same compassion as the rest. This compassion is important in view of the observation of Tait and colleagues (1990) that WCB patients face the added stress of involvement in an adversarial medicolegal system.

Mendelson (1984) compared 47 low-back-pain patients who were involved in personal injury litigation with 33 subjects without legal entanglement. On a host of psychological measures both groups scored higher on depression, neuroticism, and trait anxiety compared to the normal population. The conclusion was that involvement in litigation did not have any effect on their overall psychological profile.

Dworkin and associates (1986) in an investigation of 454 chronic pain patients demonstrated that the factor that distinguished response to treatment was employment status at the point of inception. Patients employed at the time of admission to the treatment program responded more positively to treatment than those who were not. Employment, rather than litigation or compensation, was the single most powerful predictor of outcome. In a more recent study Gallagher and colleagues (1995) investigated the characteristics of disabled persons applying for workers compensation. A total of 169 unemployed low-back pain subjects received comprehensive medical and psychological assessment. Neither compensation status nor the involvement of a lawyer improved prediction of employment status, and did not reduce the probability of return to work.

In an earlier paper, Gallagher and associates (1989) compared 87 subjects with low-back pain attending a pain clinic with 63 subjects with low-back pain who had applied for, but had not received, compensation. At the initial assessment the compensation group provided more evidence of chronicity and physical and biomechanical decompensation. These differences disappeared when the length of time out of work was taken into account. Gallagher's group concluded that exclusive reliance on physical examination along with inadequate consideration of psychological factors and adjustments for age and length of time out of work would result in an incomplete and distorted clinical picture. An inference of this study was that applying for compensation was not a signal of unwillingness to return to work.

Unfortunately, there is evidence to suggest that knowledge of a patient's compensation payment status tends to influence clinical judgment (Simmonds *et al.*, 1996). A convenience sample of 69 physical therapists viewed three video-taped assessments of patients with low-back pain that differed in severity. The subjects were provided with the compensation status of the patients: one group was receiving compensation, and the other was not. A third group of subjects was not provided with this information. The results showed that the knowledge of compensation status did not influence the subjects' physical assessment findings, but it did influence prognostic judgments. Compensation status was deemed to have a negative effect on outcome in patients with mild low-back pain, whereas noncompensation status had a positive influence on outcome in patients with severe low-back pain. This study furnishes some evidence of the built-in prejudice that we clinicians have in relation to chronic pain patients on compensation. The greatest doubt we have about these patients is their motivation to return to work. As shown in the preceding chapter, motivation appears to be prerequisite for success for returning to work.

The complexity involved in assessing depression and anxiety in a group of 201 chronic pain patients was noted by Tait and colleagues (1990). Ninety-nine patients were working, 15 were working and litigating, 3 were receiving workers compensation, and 34 were receiving workers compensation and litigating. They found that the interactions showed the effects of litigation to be mediated by work status. Litigating workers compensation patients reported less distress than nonlitigants, whereas distress levels were higher among working litigating patients than among nonlitigants. This study challenges the presupposition that being involved in litigation is necessarily distressing for our patients.

Burns and associates (1995) warned that workers compensation patients should not be considered high risks for failure solely because of their compensation status. They investigated 158 workers compensation recipients and found that subjects with high initial pain and a history of pain-related surgery fared worse than any other group. Subjects not characterized by high pain and a history of surgery responded as well as noncompensation subjects. One again, motivation in the way of pessimistic belief in the ability to return to their former occupation among the compensation subjects emerged as a significant predictor for failure.

An earlier study found support for the effectiveness of a hospital-based occupational rehabilitation program for subjects on compensation for work-related low-back injuries as opposed to the subjects who were denied such treatment by the workers compensation insurance company (Tollison, 1991). A comparison study of 44 patients with work-related low-back injuries on compensation who participated in the treatment and 20 patients who were denied treatment by their insurance company showed at the 12-month follow-up that the population of workers who participated in treatment were more likely to return to work, consumed fewer analgesics, and required fewer hospitalizations and fewer additional surgeries than those who were denied treatment. Apparently, being on compensation and treatment success are not mutually exclusive. Even common sense dictates that denial of treatment can only have negative consequences for the patients.

Summary

The research literature is almost unanimous in the general finding that motive for litigation or financial compensation arising out of injury has very little, if any, negative consequences for treatment success or for rehabilitation with the specific purpose of returning workers' compensation patients to work. There is also wide acceptance of the truth that malingering is rare and not easy to identify. The inevitable question then is, why do so many patients seeking compensation or disability benefits end up feeling frustrated and have their veracity questioned? It is an oversimplification to attribute this problem to public or private insurance companies or workers compensation boards. They rely solely on the medical opinions of independent, as well as their own, physicians for their adjudication. The case of Mrs. Inkster is instructive. The psychiatric opinion of somatoform disorder is a perfectly legitimate psychiatric condition, but, as with so many psychiatric conditions, it carries a certain amount of uncertainty with it, which in turn creates a certain amount of bias not uncommonly shared by the health care community. Another complication was the psychiatrist's observation of her behavior and demeanor which provided little or no evidence of distress associated with chronic pain. This, minimally, brings into question her claim of significant pain-related disability. The specter of malingering or partial malingering was thus raised.

Another hurdle for Mrs. Inkster was the diagnosis of fibromyalgia. This diagnosis, although increasingly recognized as a valid and potentially debilitating disorder, shares with somatoform disorder that same bias. Many health care professionals have serious questions about its legitimacy, and view this condition with much suspicion. An added problem is any kind of association between a trauma, work related or not, and fibromyalgia or somatoform disorder. In the absence of any tangible connection and if there is any evidence of predisposition, such claims are easily rejected. It would be nearly impossible to show, in our present state of knowledge, any association between Mrs. Inkster's accident and fibromyalgia. Recall that Mrs. Inkster had a past record of automobile accidents which left no lasting mark on her.

The entire relationship between workers and WCB and insurance companies tends to be adversarial. Patients often report their feeling of helplessness in the face of a powerful organization that they view as determined to deny their claim. Tait and colleagues (1990) reported that workers who engaged lawyers to fight workers compensation boards felt less anxiety than those who did not. The authors speculated that the need to retain legal counsel was promoted by the workers' perception that the adversarial proceedings would work against appropriate treatment or settlement, and retaining legal counsel would provide the claimants a modicum of protection against a powerful adversary. Mrs. Inkster had no doubt that her employers were singular in their determination to deny her disability benefits, and wondered what would convince them of her inability to work.

Since financial gain is rarely a motive for seeking disability and other financial benefits, we consider the psychological benefits that accrue from adopting the chronic sick role. *Secondary gain* is the term used to describe this phenomenon.

We shall end this discussion by quoting from the *Winnipeg Free Press* of August 27, 1999,

> For the first time, a decision by a special Manitoba panel that hears automobile injury compensation appeals has been overturned. Manitoba's top court has quashed a decision made by the Automobile Injury Compensation Appeals Commission, a panel created in 1993 to hear appeals made by accident victims who believe their compensation through no-fault insurance is inadequate.
>
> In a Court of Appeal decision written by Justice Bonnie Helper, the court ruled that the Commission was in error in supporting a Manitoba Public Insurance (MPI) decision to cut off benefits to a woman injured in a car accident ... Yesterday's ruling involved Carmen Welch, who was involved in a car accident in 1994. She was 56 at the time and working as a nursing attendant, a job in which she bathed and groomed bed-ridden patients. Welch found that she could no longer work after the accident because of pain and quit her job in November 1996.
>
> MPI ruled they would have eased Welch back into work over a period of months and agreed to pay her benefits, known as income replacement indemnity, only until March 1997, at which time benefits were terminated.
>
> Welch appealed to the Commission, which upheld MPI's decision, although it extended benefits one more month to the end of April 1997. The Appeal Court has ordered all benefits restored to Welch retroactive to the cut-off date pending further action by MPI ... The court found the Commission had no evidence on which to base its decisions in denying Welch her benefits.

This case endorses the adversarial quality of the worker–insurance company or WCB relationship, and further reinforces the need for willingness and financial resources for our patients to fight on. Many, if not most, of our patients choose not to dispute because they do not have the means. The need to replace the adversarial model with a collaborative one can hardly be overemphasized. That kind of rethinking falls squarely in the political domain, and as clinicians we have little or no power to effect such an outcome.

SECONDARY GAIN

The concept of secondary gain is rooted in the Parsonian elucidation of the sick role. The sick role bestows on the patient a number of privileges, such as suspension of duties and being cared for by others, including the medical system. Maintaining those privileges without fulfilling the obligations, another requirement of the sick role, clearly illustrates secondary gain. Chronic illness complicates the situation by removing the possibility of regaining complete health: hence the need for realignment of duties and responsibilities. Being cared for also becomes a reality for many chronic patients. Malingering and secondary gain are generally treated as the same phenomenon. For the purpose of this discussion, secondary gain is defined as an unconscious phenomenon, which has its genesis in the patient's needs to being cared for and to have emotional and psychological needs met through dependency. It can also free the patient from undesirable and unattractive chores. Secondary gain differs from malingering in one significant way. Malingering is a conscious and deliberate act to deceive, and the benefits are more often than not tangible. Benefits of secondary gain are not always evident, even to the patient. We explore this concept by discussing a case in which secondary gain seemed significant and by reviewing the literature.

This case is intriguing because the spouse of the patient played a major role in fostering the patient's helpless posture. The patient's disability extricated both parties from long-term conflict. The case involved a 39-year-old man who had emigrated to Canada from India some years ago. Despite his college education, Mr. Jain could find only menial jobs. His wife, an ambitious woman, was dissatisfied with her husband's lack of drive and "was on his case" all the time, according to the patient. Then Mr. Jain had a car accident and sustained a whiplash injury. He recovered and returned to work after a few weeks, but experienced pain in lifting and shifting. He took time off work and thus began his sojourn through the medical and other systems. When he arrived at the pain clinic, he had had extensive orthopedic and neurological investigations without any great revelations.

At our first encounter at the pain clinic, his wife acted as his spokesperson. She catalogued all the physicians "they" had visited and basically lambasted the

medical profession for its greed and lack of competence. She was no less sparing
of the WCB, who had been giving them the proverbial runaround. It was difficult
at this session to get a coherent history of the patient or the family. Mr. Jain was
invited to come back alone, which he did, and his personal history revealed his
accepting attitude to almost everything in life, which was also a major source of
his wife's criticism.

How had she reacted to his accident? She had been a tower of strength, and
he was very grateful to her for taking charge. Her attitude toward him had
changed dramatically. Instead of being critical, she became solicitous, and there
was peace in the family.

This story is remarkable, but not unusual in that an external event solved a
longstanding marital conflict. The secondary gain element is almost self-evident.
The accident extricated the patient from the pressure of improving his lot, and his
wife found a new cause which she pursued with great vigor. Mr. and Mrs. Jain
were practically in a state of war with all the major systems, and when Mr. Jain
left the pain clinic, without completing his treatment, nothing much had changed.
A case can be made that Mr. Jain's motivation for recovery and return to work
was sufficiently modified by the remarkable change in his wife's attitude toward
him. This is another facet of secondary gain which does not receive much
attention in the clinical literature. The psychological benefit accruing from illness
is the gain, and is fundamentally different from falsification or exaggeration of
symptoms for financial gain. Mrs. Jain pursued the case with WCB with much
zest. Yet these patients present a real challenge to the clinical community.
Secondary gain has different and divergent manifestations as the following review
will show. Only a careful understanding of the psychological and interpersonal
changes brought about by illness in a family member is capable of unraveling
gains that a patient or a couple or a family experiences.

It is intriguing that a similar phenomenon was reported in 1969 that linked
the etiology of traumatic and compensation neurosis with "morbid secondary
gains" (Welz, 1968–1969). A report a year later noted that the "attitudes of wife
may discourage a return to work (for her husband), in part because he releases her
from part of the load of child care" (Antibi, 1970). This last statement, as in the
case of Mr. Jain, points out the complex intrapersonal and interpersonal factors
that influence secondary gain. In contemporary behavioral literature this type of
spousal behavior is described as reinforcement of pain behaviors. These spouses
did not cause their husbands to have accidents, but the accident resolved past
conflicts either in the domain of distribution of domestic responsibilities or more
complex marital conflicts. The literature clearly points in the direction that both
physically ill patients and somatizers demonstrate secondary gain problems,
usually increased attention from family members, in equal proportion (Fishbain
et al., 1995). This observation is extraordinarily astute because, in general, much

of the literature tends to emphasize an association between secondary gain and emotional and psychiatric conditions.

The most exhaustive review to date on the topic of secondary gain is reported by Fishbain and his associates (1995). Their literature search revealed 166 references in which primary, secondary, or tertiary gain was mentioned. In relation to pain literature, they found three areas of inquiry into the secondary gain concept:

1. The sick role itself or marital reinforcement of it as an impetus to maintaining the disability;
2. Compensation (financial) as an impetus to maintaining the sick status (reviewed in the preceding section);
3. Direct investigation of the secondary gain concept.

Their general conclusion was that the secondary gain research was weak and constrained by many methodological flaws. One other conclusion was that receipt of disability benefits did not change patient behavior. They also noted that preinjury or postinjury patients did not necessarily act consciously in ways to obtain benefits.

In a complex study to determine the influence of stressful life events and secondary gains, 44 somatizers were compared with 11 subjects who had psychiatric disorders but complained only of psychological symptoms, 39 subjects who had "mixed" conditions involving independent psychiatric and physical illness, 90 patients who had physical illness, and 123 healthy members of the general population (Craig *et al.*, 1994). Somatizers were defined as subjects who had recently visited their general practitioners with physical complaints but no organic basis was found for the complaint (note the similarity with many chronic pain patients). The rating of the secondary gain potential was defined by the investigators as an attempt to estimate the likelihood that the development of a publicly declared physical illness could reverse, prevent, or lessen the undesirable consequences of the crisis, either through affording an escape from the situation or by effecting a desirable change in the social environment which could mitigate the undesirable consequences of the crisis, such as gaining monetary or other practical compensation.

The findings of this study were complex, but for our purpose the somatizers and the psychologizers were more likely to have experienced one life-event 38 weeks prior to the onset of the symptom which had the potential for secondary gain. In a two-year follow-up, subsequent functional illnesses were also associated with experiences which had secondary gain potential. One tentative conclusion of this study was that a specific relationship between a particular social experience (a crisis with potential for secondary gain) and somatization existed.

It must be noted that secondary gain was not defined necessarily as a negative attribute. The authors gave the example of a woman who was physically assaulted by her husband, left home the next day, and saw an attorney to initiate divorce proceedings. This is major departure from, and indeed an extension of, the conventional understanding of secondary gain. Nevertheless, secondary gain appears to be more commonly associated with somatizers, and given the added complexity of this concept, the question of secondary gain should be examined even with greater care with chronic pain sufferers whose pain cannot be satisfactorily explained by organic factors.

McIntosh and associates (1995) in their discussion of barriers to rehabilitation of back-injury patients noted that, in addition to lack of clear goals for rehabilitation and lack of motivation, secondary gain may also hinder rehabilitation. In their analysis secondary gain included financial and psychological gains. They did not distinguish between conscious and unconscious gains, but nevertheless recognized that both kinds of gains could hinder rehabilitation. In an earlier discussion of a comprehensive approach to dealing with idiopathic chronic pain, Brent and Flemm (1981) described a case of a 77-year-old female to show how reinforcing behaviors which promote secondary gain could be reduced. Their analysis emphasized the psychological aspect of secondary gain and the roles of the medical profession and others that help to maintain secondary gain.

"Unconscious" secondary gain was shown in a clinical study of four patients, ages 12 to 24, with conversion disorders (Schulman, 1988). The treatment was geared to reducing the secondary gain, as it might have been a powerful source to perpetuate the illness. This study also stressed the need for the whole family to be involved in the treatment. The treatment focused on encouraging the patients to cope with their ongoing responsibilities. In other words, they were discouraged from assuming the sick role.

SUMMARY

In this chapter we have made an arbitrary distinction between conscious decision to emulate pain and disability (malingering) and secondary gain, an unconscious phenomenon. We also noted that secondary gain is associated with effective coping. By and large, however, the gain is in the psychological and/or interpersonal domain. In the literature the distinction between conscious and unconscious benefits is subsumed under the concept of secondary gain. In fact, secondary gain is increasingly associated with attainment of financial rewards (Fishbain et al., 1995). Our approach is somewhat unorthodox, yet the distinction is important as it has serious consequences for treatment. There appears to be an overemphasis on malingering because of the political–legal aspect of it. Secondary gain, on the other hand, is generally overlooked because it does not directly impact the decisions related to financial compensation. Nevertheless, secondary gain, with Mr. and Mrs. Jain, may jeopardize rehabilitation, and the matter of financial compensation was, from all accounts, unresolved.

The entire problem of malingering and secondary gain will continue to remain controversial as long as the diagnostic problems associated with idiopathic chronic pain conditions remain unclear. With all the advances in pain management, a significant proportion of chronic pain patients tend to become disabled in varying degrees. The legitimacy of that disability is almost always suspect since there is rarely an objective measure of the level of disease to justify the level of disability. The level of disability associated with rheumatoid arthritis cannot be subject to the same kind of subjectivity as fibromyalgia or even worse, chronic low-back pain of unknown origin. Hence, the difficulties that our patients encounter when filing a compensation claim are not likely to be resolved in the foreseeable future. One solution requires an attitude change about malingering by the WCB and employers, based on the knowledge that malingering is rare. Thus, from the beginning of the process, our patients will not be viewed with suspicion.

When there is no clear or acceptable medical diagnosis, the patient's veracity may be questioned and an underlying psychiatric problem may be assumed. The conceptualization of chronic pain over the last two or more decades has moved away from the strict Cartesian duality of body and mind. A biopsychosocial formulation of the problem is widely accepted, and most pain management clinics operate on integrative principles. However, when a psychiatric opinion is sought by an insurance company, it is not to legitimize a patient's claim but to dismiss it. In the case of Mrs. Inkster, the psychiatrist raised the possibility of masked depression. The entire question of pain and depression has received an inordinate amount of scrutiny in the literature, and the general consensus is that masked depression may not be a viable diagnosis for chronic pain conditions.

We see that a questionable diagnosis, such as masked depression, raises suspicion about the patient's condition. We address physicians' attitudes to chronic pain in the next chapter. It is more than conceivable that many of our patients will continue to feel powerless by their encounter with powerful employers and WCB.

Chapter 10

THE PATIENT AND THE MEDICAL WORLD: MRS. KRAMER'S JOURNEY THROUGH THE MEDICAL SYSTEM

INTRODUCTION

Pain clinics are often the last line of defense for treatment of chronic nonbenign pain which did not respond to medical intervention. The patients there have been often disappointed, and they have a small hope that they may find some relief. Some arrive quite angry with the medical profession: "They can send people to the moon, but can't cure my headache" is a statement this author has heard more than once. Their anger is obviously due to lack of resolution of the pain problem. Another reason is their growing sense that many physicians question the veracity of their pain complaint, and the inference that the pain is more in their head (which makes them wonder if they are crazy) than organic. We shall examine some factors that might contribute to the patient's disillusionment with health care professionals. We describe in detail a patient's journey through the health care system which shows the necessity of the investigations that patients have to endure and provides insight into the patient's growing frustration and loss of trust in the medical profession to find a reasonable solution to their debilitating pain.

MRS. KRAMER ON THE MEDICAL TREADMILL

We chose Mrs. Kramer because she had kept a detailed account of her journey through the medical system. She also had all her medical reports. In addition, we interviewed her on tape for an hour and a half, and she described the lengthy and sometimes unpleasant encounter with the health care system and, in particular, physicians.

Mrs. Kramer, 55 years old, was referred to our pain clinic with chronic low-back pain, secondary osteoarthritis with a large muscular component, and spinal stenosis. She was married and had a married daughter and a granddaughter. Her family situation was stable. She and her husband emigrated to Canada from Eastern Europe some 35 years ago, obtained suitable employment, and led the good life they had expected. Her job was in the financial sector, and she stayed with the firm for over 25 years as a senior clerk dealing with payments and invoices until she could no longer work due to her pain problems. Her husband was kind and considerate, but had his own health problems. Just before her most recent health problem, they were considering retiring and just enjoying themselves. Mrs. Kramer, after her pain began sought long-term disability, which was the beginning of her "prolonged period of humiliation and disappointment." Note that Mrs. Kramer is a highly intelligent, cultured woman with an excellent command of English.

Her back pain began in 1978, at which time she received physiotherapy and was put in an orthopedic corset. She recalled the events: "At the end of 1978 they put me in a body cast because my posture was very crooked and I was unable to walk straight. After that I was able to cope with the back problem till 1987, which means that occasionally I spent a weekend in bed. I go to work and straight from work I go home to bed. I was trying to exercise to get my health back." She was off work for a few weeks, and her pain problem remained essentially dormant for 10 years. Also in 1978, she had surgery for malignant melanoma and was off work for 10 days. The surgery was successful, and other than an occasional feeling of trepidation about its recurrence, Mrs. Kramer emerged relatively unscathed from this experience. To this point her experience of the health care system and her physicians was altogether positive. She admitted that she had an "old country" attitude of great respect for the medical profession.

In 1987, Mrs. Kramer's back problem worsened, and she had surgery to remove vertebral spurs. The surgery was again successful, and she returned to work after three months of rehabilitation and recuperation. She stated: "In 1987 they recommended back surgery because I had bulging discs and also bone spurs. After the surgery I was home for three months and after that I went back to work. I was taking medication and doing physiotherapy. I was going swimming twice a week. I had a very scheduled life, but I was able to carry on." In retrospect, this episode was the turning point, and the beginning of her chronic pain problem. Despite the success of the surgery, she began to experience more diffused pain in various parts of her body. It was not debilitating, and she was able to live normally.

In 1994 she was diagnosed with fibromyalgia by her family physician. The diagnosis gave her some comfort as well as rationale for her pain, but changed little in terms of management of it. She knew nothing about fibromyalgia, but she had great faith in her physician. He referred her to a specialist in physical medicine, who helped her control her muscle spasms and improve her sleep. For the next two years she was under the care of a physical medicine specialist. But to her great dismay, her family physician of 26 years left for the United States in 1997.

She had many difficulties in finding another physician, mainly because not many family physicians were accepting new patients, and she wanted her physician within a reasonable distance from home. Finally she found a family physician, whom she liked a great deal, but he left for the United States only after a year or two, and Mrs. Kramer was again on the lookout for a family physician. She recalled: "After my doctor left for America, I had to look for a new doctor again. I had three or four days to find a new doctor who was taking new patients. There was one doctor who was taking new patients, but he was working only two days a week. The wait to see him was three to four weeks. I knew that I needed someone more accessible. So I finally found a young doctor who was very confident and his clinic was close to my house."

The departure of her family physician coincided with increasing back pain. Her muscle spasms returned and she developed severe muscle-contraction-type headaches. By the end of 1997, any movement of her legs caused excruciating pain. She was placed on Tylenol 3 by her new family physician and scheduled for a CT scan. She was off work for five days at the end of 1997. She also started physiotherapy, but discontinued it after three weeks because it aggravated her pain.

She was concerned about becoming dependent on codeine. She also sought her physician's guidance about a vacation in the southern United States. While on vacation, her general health improved and her pain decreased to the point that she felt reasonably functional. She returned to work but within a week her back pain became quite severe. She was told to take one Tylenol 3 every four hours. Her sleep pattern became disturbed and she complained of lack of concentration and fatigue. Only two weeks after returning from vacation, she had to go on sick leave.

In March 1998 she had a CT scan, which revealed some degenerative changes. She was referred to a neurosurgeon by her family physician. The neurosurgeon conducted more tests and concluded that surgery was not needed. However, she had a bone scan which showed abnormalities of the spine, but these were attributed to simple degenerative changes.

Between October 1998 and her referral to the pain clinic in March 1999, she saw a neurosurgeon, a physiatrist, an oncologist, a cardiologist, and a rheumatologist. In October 1998 her third family physician left, and again she had to find a replacement. In March 1999, she was referred to a pain clinic. Just before entering the pain clinic, she had a comprehensive medical examination by an independent physician to assess her eligibility for Canada Pension (Disability). He offered the following diagnoses in rank order:

1. Chronic pain disorder
2. Depression

3. Fibromyalgia syndrome
4. Mechanical low-back pain most likely due to degenerative changes
5. Myofascial pain syndrome (very mild)

He further noted that Mrs. Kramer had at least a sedentary work capacity and suggested modifications to make the job more suitable to her medical condition. She never worked again.

At some point in her suffering her attitude to medicine in general and physicians in particular began to change. Her most prominent feeling was that many physicians failed to appreciate her level of pain and incapacity or simply did not believe her. Her change of attitude was not simply a matter of physicians becoming unsympathetic to her or treating her with disrespect. This issue was complicated by at least three factors:

1. Her own disappointment with the ineffectual treatment for her pain
2. Physicians' frustration in dealing with a patient who was not only unresponsive to treatment but often presented with new problems
3. The patient finding herself in total disagreement with the independent physician's assessment of her work capacity.

There was also a fourth factor, which involved the patient being passed, not for trivial reasons, from one specialty to the next, none of which was particularly helpful. Thus, in Mrs. Kramer's mind the medical profession had no idea about what to do with her or was simply passing her along to someone else to tell her again there was not much wrong with her. She began questioning her sanity. Was she imagining her pain? Was it all in her head? Was there medical cause for her pain? Mrs. Kramer's experience with the medical system is summarized here:

1978	First experience of back pain: physiotherapy; orthopedic corset
1978	Malignant melanoma: surgery
1987	Back surgery: removal of vertebral spurs
1994	Diagnosed with fibromyalgia by family physician
1994	First contact with physiatrist: lasted two years
1997 June	Departure of her long-time family physician
1997 Dec.	New family physician treats her with Tylenol 3 for worsening pain; CT scan ordered
1998 Jan.	Physiotherapy commenced, but soon discontinued due to increasing discomfort
1998 Feb.	Pain worsens; medication increased; stops work
1998 March	CT scan
1998 March	Eye problem: new eyeglasses
1998 March	CT scan showed problems: sees neurosurgeon

1998 July	Myelogram and another CT scan; surgery not recommended
1998 Aug.	Emergency visit due to a fall; sprained ankle
1998 Sept.	Bone scan: number of abnormalities involving the spine
1998 Oct.	Family physician leaves practice: new family physician takes over
1998 Oct.	X-ray of thoracic spine; no positive findings
1998 Nov.	Oncologist for annual checkup; scan of thoracic spine; widespread degenerative changes
1999 Jan.	Independent medical examination for disability pension
1999 Jan.	MRI test; returns to physiatrist; sees a clinical psychologist
1999 Feb.	Sees cardiologist concerning rapid heart beat: stress test and is placed on anti-hypertensive drug
1999 Feb.	Sees neurosurgeon
1999 March	Seen at pain clinic
1999 April	Stress test
1999 June	Sees rheumatologist
1999 Nov.	Continues to be a patient at the pain clinic. Medical treadmill stops

Literature Review

To what extent could Mrs. Kramer's feelings of physicians' perceived or real frustration with her be attributed to their attitude to chronic illness in general and chronic pain in particular? A paper written in 1932 described in great detail the attitude a patient should take toward his or her doctor. The three most salient principles related to the patient's attitude were that (1) the person should talk freely with the physician; (2) the physician should give the patient the *impression* that he or she is there to help, and is doing everything possible; and (3) the family should show a cooperative attitude toward the patient. There is, of course, a great deal of variability in a patient's attitude to the physician, and vice versa. It is nonetheless clear that the patient should share all pertinent information with the physician (Stevenson, 1932). This is true at all times.

The second proposition demands attention. Physicians were expected to only give the impression that they were interested in their patients. One of the common complaints our patients have about their interaction with many physicians is their lack of sympathy for the patient's intractable pain. A recent study that examined the relationship between physicians and patients suffering from chronic fatigue syndrome found that patients were satisfied with medical care if only their expectations were consistent with the medical system (Twemlow *et al.*, 1997). This study further confirmed that chronic fatigue syndrome patients had a generally more negative attitude toward the medical profession.

In relation to chronic pain patients, expectations rarely coincide with the medical system because the pain itself often remains impervious to the medical ministrations. This last point is the center of patient–physician hostility. The source of this anger and disappointment is the inability of the medical profession to ameliorate the pain and the tendency to resort to psychiatric formulation in the absence of organic causes that may explain the pain. To have to live with ongoing pain and be labeled psychiatric, which is interpreted by many patients as a sign of their lack of credibility, is considered doubly insulting. Many years ago Berlin (1954) observed that many patients with psychosomatic disorders referred to psychiatrists by internists simply failed to show up or did not return after the first session. Berlin concluded that referral to psychiatry often came as a last resort, and, more significantly, many patients regarded the referral as a clear sign of rejection by the internists. Many pain patients today regard any suggestion that the cause of the pain is psychological and not organic as a clear indication of rejection or name calling by their family physician or other specialist.

The problem may not be one of resistance to psychiatry but rather to how this matter is presented. If stated in the right context—that is, the cause of the pain is unknown, but the suffering is significant and a psychiatrist might be of help—it may be more acceptable to many patients. We use a similar explanation to engage our patients in family therapy. Basically, we convince them that the pain problem is also causing significant disruption in the family system, and while all is being done to find solutions to the pain we should not ignore the family issues. Most patients accept this explanation. Their pain complaint is not marginalized or mini-mized, and they are able to appreciate the incidental problems arising out of their pain and disability.

The attitude of physicians to psychosocial problems was reported in a study of 63 medical residents (Eisenthal et al., 1994). The subjects' attitudes to psychosocial problems were, on the whole, positive but qualified. Most of these physicians were not defensive about asking personal questions without feeling nosey or believing they were interfering. The subjects also perceived the patients to be receptive to psychosocial questioning, and yet half the physicians felt that the patients were resistant to psychosocial attribution, and half the physicians indicated that the patients needed prompting to talk about life problems. The strongest influence on attitude was the setting, ambulatory care over in-patient. This is instructive for several reasons. First, physicians generally displayed positive attitudes to the exploration of psychosocial problems. While they displayed a certain reservation, the patients were resistant. The main point of this study is that a physician's attitude in itself is not a serious problem. Nevertheless, when a negative attitude to psychosocial problems is combined with resistant patients, the only possible outcome is oversight of serious social and interpersonal issues and perpetuation of a hostile attitude, mostly on the part of the patients.

On the other hand, there is some evidence to show that many physicians display negative attitudes to certain problems. This was borne out in a survey of orthopedic and neurosurgeons on the prevalence of malingering in their practices (Leavitt and Sweet, 1986). Exaggeration of symptoms and incongruity between the patient's complaint and an objective medical finding were the two dimensions commonly employed by the physicians to diagnose malingering. Malingering seemed to occur at about a 5% level according to 60% of the respondents. However, 15% of the sample reported malingering at over 20% in their practices. Malingering was considered common by one fifth of the respondents. This study begins to explain the frustration of physicians in dealing with chronic pain patients for whom the question of diagnoses is moot. It is, therefore, not altogether unpredictable that so many of our patients express such negative experiences in describing their interaction with physicians. In one way or another these patients come to believe that their pain complaints are totally dismissed or minimized such that their own veracity becomes an issue. Recall that Mrs. Kramer's pain complaints were considered valid, but her inability to return to work was interpreted as resistance. Hence, she was exaggerating her pain-related disability. Malingering was never invoked, but it remained a background issue.

Lieff (1982) argued that physicians demonstrated an avoidance toward several groups: the dying, the elderly, and the handicapped. These attitudes have significantly changed, but some of Leiff's observations remain relevant. One attitude was a feeling of helplessness when faced with seemingly unsolvable problems. This remains true of chronic pain sufferers. Even those of us who work exclusively with this population cannot deny outright the feeling of helplessness experienced in the face of a truly intractable problem, and among the chronic pain population intractable problems abound. It is more than conceivable that a person of Mrs. Kramer's sensitivity would have picked up these subtle, or perhaps not so subtle, attitudes on the part of one or two physicians. In fact, she voiced this very sentiment at the end of her medical evaluation for disability. The message she heard was: "Go back to work and all will be well." She could not go back to work, and all was not well.

In a study of doctor–patient relationships, 62 outpatients participated in a project to explore the impact of this relationship beyond patient compliance (Hezsen-Klemens and Lapinska, 1984). Two visits of every subject to the doctor were recorded. The treatment results were evaluated by physicians. It was found that the doctors' directness, their emotional attitude toward the patients, the patients' activity, and the patients' partnership status affected the patients' behavior, such as compliance with doctors' orders and the subjects' spontaneous health activity. The outcome studies of pain clinics show that a high percentage of pain patients benefits from treatment at multidisciplinary pain clinics. It is more than conceivable that the clinicians' unquestioning attitude toward their pain complaints plays a significant role in the rehabilitation of the patients. One of the first tasks of the pain clinic staff is to reassure the patient that the pain is legitimate, and then to help extricate the patient from the tiresome and mostly fruitless body–mind dichotomy, since many, if not most, of our patients have been led to believe that the pain is imaginary or in their heads.

A more recent study on physician knowledge and attitude about cancer pain found that medical specialty was the strongest influence on knowledge and attitudes, with primary care physicians having significantly better outcomes than surgeons or medical subspecialists (Elliott *et al.*, 1995). Physicians who had personal experience with cancer pain in a friend or family had more favorable attitude scores than those who did not. Mrs. Kramer's experience with her family physicians was generally favorable. However, the medical subspecialties that she encountered left her less than satisfied. The question of physician attitude is raised over and over again by many patients. Mrs. Kramer's observation was that many physicians not only did not truly appreciate her level of suffering, but through words and actions managed to trivialize her pain complaints.

Mrs. Kramer's Self-Doubt Concerning Pain Legitimacy

Pain of unknown etiology has a long and tortured history. Such pain has usually been assigned several psychiatric diagnoses. These diagnoses did not necessarily lead to treatment. In fact, such a diagnosis was almost a guarantee for no further treatment. In short, psychiatric diagnoses were a simple way to reject any organic basis for the pain. That state of affairs has changed significantly over the last two decades. Generally speaking, most pain clinics subscribe to the multidimensional nature of pain, and psychological and medical treatments are combined to maximize the benefits of treatment.

Depression is not uncommon in the chronic pain population. Of course, not so long ago chronic pain of unknown etiology was variously described as masked depression, depression without depression, a variant of a depressive disorder, and so on. There now is some consensus in the literature that a proportion of pain patients indeed suffer from clinical depression and many from dysthymia. We now examine in detail the dynamics behind Mrs. Kramer's depression and the process through which she began to believe that physicians did not fully appreciate her pain and suffering and might have suggested that her pain was "in her head."

Mrs. Kramer had seen the following specialists: orthopedic surgeon, neurosurgeon, rheumatologist, physiatrist, psychologist, cardiologist (for high heart rate), and oncologist (annual checkup). The first four specialists were directly related to her chronic pain. She had received similar messages from all four, which essentially meant that there was nothing they could do for her pain, and it was time for her to get on with her life. Recall that Mrs. Kramer's negative view of the medical profession was birthed by the discrepancy between her perceived level of disability and the "objective" medical conclusion that, although she had fibromyalgia, mechanical low-back pain, myofascial pain syndrome (mild), and depression, these conditions did not explain her level of disability. Hence, she must be exaggerating her symptoms.

At this point we wish to review her feeling of rejection or dismissal by her physicians. From her point of view, by the end of 1997 her health had deteriorated to a point that she was barely functional. Not surprisingly, this prompted a variety of medical investigations that included myelogram, CT scan, bone scan, and numerous visits to doctors and clinics. Findings from the various investigations, at least in part, justified her pain but not the associated disability. Surgery was not recommended. She was relieved about not having surgery, and she remained hopeful that ways would be found to combat her pain. It was about this time that her eyesight deteriorated so that she could no longer read. This problem was resolved, but the experience had left her even more anxious and frightened. Lack of progress with her pain condition made her tense and angry and, above all, feeling hopeless. She had many classic symptoms of depression, such as lowering of mood, poor sleep, loss of appetite, poor concentration, lack of enjoyment, and very low energy. However, many of these symptoms could be accounted for by her ever-present pain and fibromyalgia.

Depression, lack of congruity between her pain complaints and objective medical findings, her "unwillingness" to return to work, and seemingly adapting to chronic patienthood were sufficient justification from the medical point of view to raise issues about the legitimacy of her pain-related disability. One physician noted: "I cannot with 100% medical certainty identify any event in the patient's history or examination that could be clearly identified as the cause of her perceived ongoing disabling symptoms." Mrs. Kramer had no defense against such a scientific and objective observation other than to feel slighted and dismissed. The message once again was: "There isn't much wrong with you. Pull up your socks and get on with it."

Concerning depression, a *prima facie* case can be made that given the magnitude of her loss, her mood is understandable. In Mrs. Kramer we had a highly functioning human being, who made a good life for herself and her family, raised a daughter, worked for many years, overcame cancer and many episodes of back pain. For her to have a profound sense of loss for all that she valued could even be viewed as normal. In short, her mood was congruent with her situation.

To what extent did her effort to seek a disability pension play a role in maintaining her symptoms? The question of disability pension and its role in prompting Mrs. Kramer to adopt a helpless position is moot. As the evidence in an earlier chapter pointed out, malingering is rare, and yet her behavior suggested such a possibility. Once she learned that her application for disability was denied, could we have expected to see any change in her behavior, such as further worsening of her condition? The answer has to be no. At the pain clinic she received a variety of medical, psychological, and psychosocial interventions. If anything, her condition was showing signs of improvement. She was reengaging in a variety of activities and, more importantly, regaining her sense of enjoyment. She also decided not to appeal the denial of disability pension but to take early retirement. These behaviors do not add up to malingering.

SUMMARY

We have tried to explore one patient's experience with the medical world. One major problem, namely, the patient's perception of dismissiveness of the pain problem by many physicians, clearly emanates from poor communication between physicians and patients. Patients are given to misinterpretations, and many physicians tend to err on the side of brevity. It is more than a matter of curiosity that so many chronic pain sufferers experience such a high level of frustration with the medical profession. It was clear listening to Mrs. Kramer that her interpretation of physicians challenging the veracity of the severity of her pain complaint was not based on one physician making such an outrageous statement. Rather she was responding to the general statement that many physicians are likely to make in the absence of objective findings or nominal findings that may not explain the level of disability. How these types of findings are communicated are of utmost importance. Often patients are told that there is either nothing wrong with them, or that something is wrong but is nothing to worry about. This was Mrs. Kramer's experience with a neurosurgeon, who informed her that she did not require surgery and left the matter at that. Her interpretation was that he was dismissive of her condition. Perhaps a brief explanation that although she did not require neurosurgery (good news) she still had her pain to contend with might have minimized or eliminated any misunderstanding. Acknowledging the patient's suffering may go a long way to assuage that patient's negative attitudes and disappointments.

The family physician in this respect is pivotal. Since all our patients have family physicians, who generally coordinate patient care, they can and do act as the mediator between the specialist and the patient. We deal with many family physicians, and their patients tend to emerge from their journey through the medical system relatively unscathed. All information is filtered through the family physician, who has first-hand knowledge of the patient and is in a good position to communicate to the patient the findings and their implications and future plans. Communication of complicated clinical findings and their implications are of utmost importance, and again the family physician is in the best position to do that. Mrs. Kramer, for example, was unaware of the implications of having fibromyalgia. No one explained to her that sleep disturbance was a common symptom and that anti-depressants were a common treatment. Part of her problem was that in a relatively short time, she lost three family physicians. Ineffective communication under those circumstances may not be uncommon. Another factor that contributes to a patient's misunderstanding is the high level of anxiety that visits to the specialists often provoke. In such a heightened state of arousal, patients often hear what they want to hear and usually misunderstand the information received.

In conclusion, much patient suffering that seems to emanate from poor or ineffectual communication between physicians and chronic pain patients can be alleviated simply by specialists avoiding telling these patients that on the basis of their investigations there is "nothing" wrong with them. Instead they should tell them that they are unable to explain the pain. The point is that the pain is not marginalized, and the suffering of these patients is acknowledged.

A critical question has been raised here, but not answered. If Mrs. Kramer had not sought a disability pension, would her overall experience of the medical world have been different? Perhaps to a certain extent. Her family physician who diagnosed fibromyalgia either did not explain the nature of this condition or Mrs. Kramer did not comprehend the information. Similarly, her encounters with the neurosurgeon and physiatrist were not positive. It has to be acknowledged that she found the independent medical examination particularly harrowing, and it was in this situation that she felt her credibility as a patient was seriously challenged. The medical examiner did acknowledge her pain problems. However, there was such a wide gulf between the medical decision that she could return to work with some modification and her subjective state of pain and disability that she had few options in terms of what she felt about this encounter. Her feelings were independent of the physician's behavior. Disappointment can be, and often is, a major source of hopelessness, anger, and hostility.

REFERENCES

Aaromaa, M., Rautava, P., Helenius, H., and Sillanpaeae, M. (1998). Factors of early life as predictors of headache in children at school entry. *Headache*, 38, 23–30.

Ahern, D., Adams, A., and Follick, M. (1985). Emotional and marital disturbance in spouses of chronic low-back pain patients. *Clinical Journal of Pain*, 1, 69–74.

Ahern, D., and Follick, M. (1985). Distress in spouses of chronic pain patients. *International Journal of Family Therapy*, 7, 247–257.

Ahlberg-Hulten, G., and Theorell, T. (1995). Social support, job-strain and musculo-skeletal pain among female health care personnel. *Scandinavian Journal of Work, Environment and Health*, 21, 435–439.

Antibi, R. (1970). State benefits as a cause of unwillingness to work. *British Journal of Psychiatry*, 117, 205–206.

Aranson, K. (1997). Quality of life among persons with multiple sclerosis and their caregivers. *Neurology*, 48, 74–80.

Armistead, L., Klein, K., and Forehand, R. (1995). Parental physical illness and child functioning. *Clinical Psychology Review*. 15, 409–422.

Averill, P., Novy, D., Nelson, D., and Berry, L. (1996). Correlates of depression in chronic pain patients: A comprehensive examination. *Pain*. 65, 93–100.

Bar-Tal, Y. (1994). Uncertainty and the perception of sufficiency of social support, control, and information. *Psychological Record*, 44, 13–24.

Basolo-Kunzer, M., Diamond, S., and Reed, J. (1991). Chronic headache patients' marital and family adjustment. *Issues in Mental Health Nursing*, 12, 133–148.

Beardslee, W., Keller, M., and Klerman, G. (1985). Children of parents with affective disorder. *International Journal of Family Psychiatry*, 6, 283–299.

Bebbington, P., and Delemos, I. (1996). Pain in the family (Editorial). *Journal of Psychosomatic Research*, 40, 451–456.

Benjamin, S., Mawer, J., and Lennon, S. (1992). The knowledge and beliefs of family caregivers about chronic pain patients. *Journal of Psychosomatic Research*, 36, 211–217.

Berg, M. (1987). Patient education and the physician–patient relationship. *Journal of Family Practice*. 24,169–172.

Berger, H., Honig, P., and Lieberman, R. (1977). Gaining control of the symptom. *American Journal of Diseases in Children*, 131, 1340–1344.

Berlin, I. (1954). Some reasons for failures in referrals for psychiatric care of patients with psychosomatic illnesses. *Annals of Internal Medicine*, 40, 1165–1168.

Birtchnell, J., and Kennard, J. (1983). Marriage and mental illness. *British Journal of British Psychiatry*, 142, 193–198.

Bishop, D., Epstein, N., Keitner, G., Miller, I., and Srinivasan, S. (1986). Stroke: Morale, family functioning, health status and function capacity. *Archives of Physical Medicine and Rehabilitation*, 67, 84–87.

Block, A. (1981). The investigation of the response of the spouses to chronic pain behavior. *Psychosomatic Medicine*, 43, 415–422.

Blomkvist, V., Hannerz, J., Orth-Gomer, K., and Theorell, T. (1997). Coping styles and social support in women suffering from cluster headaches or migraine. *Psychotherapy and Psychosomatics*, 66, 150–154.

Bolten, W., Kempel, W., and Pforringer, W. (1998). Analyses of the cost of illness in backache. *Medizinishe Klinik*, 15, 388–393.

Bookwala, J., and Schulz, R. (1996). Spousal similarity in subjective well-being: The cardiovascular study. *Psychology and Aging*, 11, 582–590.

Borenstein, D. (1995). Epidemiology, etiology, diagnostic evaluation, and treatment of low back pain. *Current Opinion, Rheumatology*, 7, 141–146.

Brady, E. (1997). Support afforded by wives of post-myocardial infarction patients. In: Haberman, G. (Editor), *Looking back and moving forward: 50 years of New Zealand psychology*. Wellington, NZ: New Zealand Psychological Society.

Brent, R., and Flamm, G. (1981). The management of idiopathic chronic pain: A holistic approach. *Canadian Journal of Psychiatry*, 26, 429–431.

Brodarty, H., and Luscombe, G. (1998). Psychological morbidity in caregivers with depression in patients with dementia. *Alzheimer Disease and Associated Disorders*, 12, 62–70.

Brown, G., and Harris, T. (1978). *Social origin of depression*. London: Tavistock.

Brown, G., Wallston, K., and Nicassio, P. (1989). Social support and depression in rheumatoid arthritis: A one year prospective study. *Journal of Applied Social Psychology*, 19, 1164–1181.

Buck, R., and Hohnmann, G. (1982). Child adjustment as related to severity of parental disability. *Archives of Physical Medicine and Rehabilitation*, 63, 249–253.

Burns, J., Johnson, B., Mahoney, N. and Devine, J. (1996). Anger management style, hostility and spouse responses: gender differences in predictions of adjustment among chronic pain patients. *Pain*, 64, 445–453.

Burns, J., Sherman, M., Devine, J., and Mahoney, N. (1995). Association between workers' compensation and outcome following multidisciplinary treatment for chronic pain. *Clinical Journal of Pain*, 11, 94–102.

Campbell, T., and Patterson, J. (1995). The effectiveness of family intervention in the treatment of physical illness. *Journal of Marital and Family Therapy*, 21, 545–583.

Caplan, G. (1981). Mastery of stress: Psychological aspects. *American Journal of Psychiatry*, 138, 413–420.

Carosella, A., Lackner, J., and Feuerstein, M. (1994). Factors associated with early discharge from a multi-disciplinary work-rehabilitation program for chronic low back pain. *Pain*, 57, 69–76.

Carter, R., and Carter, C. (1994). Marital adjustment and effects of illness in married pairs with one or both spouses chronically ill. *American Journal of Family Therapy*, 22, 315–326.

Charles, M., and Hopflinger, F. (1992). Gender, culture and the division of labor: A replication of US studies for the case of Switzerland. *Journal of Comparative Family Studies*, 23, 375–387.

Christensen, D. (1983). Post-mastectomy couple counselling: An outcome study of a structured treatment protocol. *Sex and Marriage Therapy*, 9, 266–275.

Chun, D., Turner, J., and Romano, J. (1993). Children of chronic pain patients: Risk factors for maladjustment. *Pain*. 52, 311–317.

Clarkin, J., Glick, I., Hass, G., Spence, J., Lewis, A., Peyser, A., DeMane, A., Good-Ellis, M., Harris, M., and Lestelle, V. (1990). A randomized clinical trial of in-patient family intervention: Result of affective disorders. *Journal of Affective Disorders*, 18, 17–28.

Claussen, A. (1981). Marital role, life-stage and response to mental illness. American Sociological Association Paper.

Claussen, B., Bjorndal, A., and Hjort, P. (1993). Health and re-employment in a two-year follow-up of long-term unemployed. *Journal of Epidemiology and Community Health*. 47,14–18.

Clemmer, D., and Mohr, D. (1991). Low-back injuries in heavy industry. *Spine*. 16, 831–834.

Colom, F., Vieta, E., Martinez, A., Jorquera, A., and Gasto, C. (1998). What is the role of psychotherapy in the treatment of bipolar disorder? *Psychotherapy and Psychosomatics*, 67, 3–9.

Commission on the Evaluation of Pain (1987). Report of the Commission on the evaluation of pain. *Social Science Bulletin*, 50/1, 13–44.

Comstock, G., and Hesling, K. (1976). Symptoms of depression in two communities. *Journal of Abnormal Psychology*, 6, 551–563.

Cook, A., and Roy, R. (1995.). Attitudes, beliefs and illness behavior. In: Roy, R. (Editor), *Chronic pain in old age*. Toronto: University of Toronto Press.

Craig, T., Drake, H., Mills, K., and Boardman, A. (1994). The South London somatization study II: The influence of stressful life events and secondary gain. *British Journal of Psychiatry*, 165, 245–258.

Craig, K., Hill, M., and McMurty, B. (1998). Detecting deception and malingering. In: Block, A., Kremer, E., and Fernandez, E. (Editors). *Handbook of pain syndromes: Biopsychosocial perspective*. Mahwah, NJ: Lawrence Erlbaum Associates.

Creed, F., and Ash, G. (1992). Depression in rheumatoid arthritis: Aetiology and treatment. *International Review of Psychiatry*, 4, 23–33.

Cronan, T., Hay, M., Groessl, E., Bigatti, S., Gallagher, R., and Tomita, M. (1998). The effects of social support and education on health care costs after three years. *Arthritis Care and Research*, 11, 326–334.

Culpan, R., and Taylor, C. (1973). Psychiatric disorders following road traffic and industrial injuries. *Australian and New Zealand Journal of Psychiatry*, 7, 32–39.

D'Arcy, C., and Siddique, C. (1987). Unemployment and health: an analysis of "Canada Health Survey" data. *International Journal Health Services*, 15, 609–635.

Deardorff, W., Rubin, H., and Scott, D. (1991). Comprehensive multidisciplinary treatment of chronic pain: A follow-up study of treated and non-treated groups. *Pain*, 45, 35–43.

De Mulder, E., Tarulla, L., Kilmer-Dougan, B., Free, K., et al. (1985). Personality disorders of affectively ill mothers: Links to maternal behavior. *Journal of Personality Disorder*, 9, 199–212.

DeRiddler, D., and Schreurs, K. (1996). Coping, social support and chronic disease: A research agenda. *Psychology, Health and Medicine*, 1, 71–82.

Dew, M., Bromet, E., and Penkower, L. (1992). Mental Health effects of job loss in women. *Psychological Medicine*. 22, 751–764.

Dickstein, S., Seifor, R., Hagolen, L., Schiller, M., Sameroff, A., Keitnor, G., Miller, I., Rasmussen, S., Malzko, M., and Magee, K. (1998). Ll Levels of family assessment: Impact of maternal psychopathology on family functioning. *Journal of Family Psychology*. 12, 23–40.

Doeglas, D., Suurmeyer, T., Krol, B., and Sanderman, R. (1994). Social support, social disability, and psychological well-being in rheumatoid arthritis. *Arthritis Care and Research*, 7, 10–15.

Dooley, D., Fielding, J., and Levi, L. (1996). Health and Unemployment, *Annual Review of Public Health*, 17, 449–465.

Dozios, D., Dobson, V., Wong, M., and Hughes, D. (1995). Factors associated with rehabilitation outcome in patients with low back pain: Prediction of employment outcome at 9 month follow-up. *Rehabilitation Psychology*, 40, 243–256.

Dreiser, R., Maheu, E., Ahozlan, R., Rozenberg, S., Bourgeot, P., Bregeon, C., Benha-mou, C., Sobert, J., and Treves, R. (1997). An epidemiological study of diagnos-tic and therapeutic strategies in office practice patients with sub-acute or chronic pain in the thoracic or low-back pain. Comparison of practices in primary care or rheumatology setting. *Review of Rheumatology*, English Edition, 64, 26–34.

Dura, J., and Beck, S. (1988). A comparison of family functions when mothers have chronic pain. *Pain*. 35, 79–89.

Dworkin, R., Richlin, D., Handlin, D., and Brand, L. (1986). Predicting treatment response in depressed and non-depressed chronic pain patients. *Pain*, 24, 49–59.

Eales, M. (1988). Depression and anxiety in unemployed men. *Psychological Medi-cine*, 18, 935–945.

Eisenthal, S., Stoeckle, J., and Ehrilch, C. (1994). Orientation of medical residents to the psychosocial aspects of primary care: Influence of training program. *Academic Medicine*, 69, 48–54.

Ektor, A., Janzon, L., and Sjiland, B. (1992). Chronic pain and socioeconomic environment. Results from the pain clinic at Malmo General Hospital in Sweden. *Clinical Journal of Pain*, 9, 183–188.

Elliott, T., Murray, D., Elliott, B., and Bran, B. (1995). Physicians knowledge and attitudes about cancer pain management: A survey from the Minnesota cancer pain project. *Journal of Pain Symptom Management*, 10, 495–504.

Engel C., Von Korff, M., and Kation, W. (1996). Back in primary care: Predictors of high health care costs. *Pain*: 65, 197–204.

Epstein, N., and Bishop, D. (1981). Problem-centred systems family therapy. In Gurman, A., and Khiskeon, D. (Editors). *Handbook of Family Therapy*. New York: Brunner/Hazel.

Epstein, N., Bishop, D., and Baldwin, L. (1981). McMaster model of family functioning: A view of the normal family. In: Watch, F. (Editor). *Normal family processes*. New York: Guilford, pp. 115–141.

Epstein, N., Bishop, D., Keitner, G., and Miller, I. (1988). Combined use of pharmacological and family therapy. In: Clarkin, J., Hass, G., and Glick, I. (Editors). *Affective disorders and the family: Assessment and treatment*. New York: Guilford. pp. 153–172.

Evers, A., Kraaimaat, F., Geenen, R., and Bijlsma, J. (1997). Determinants of psychological distress and its course in the first year after diagnosis of rheumatoid arthritis. *Journal of Behavioral Medicine*, 20, 489–504.

Ewart, C., Taylor, C., Kraemer, H., and Aragas, W. (1984). Reducing blood pressure reactivity during interpersonal conflict: Effects of marital communication training. *Behaviour Therapy*, 15, 473–484.

Feuerstein, M., Sult, S., and Houle, M. (1985). Environmental stressors and chronic low-back pain: Life-events, family and work environment. *Pain*. 22, 295–307.

Finerman, R., and Bennett, L. (1995). Overview: Guilt, blame and shame in sicknesses. *Social Science and Medicine*, 40, 1–3.

Fishbain, D., Rosomoff, H., Cutler, R., and Rosomoff, R. (1995). Secondary gain concept: A review of the scientific evidence. *Clinical Journal of Pain*, 11, 16–21.

Fitzpatrick, R., Newman, S., Lamb, R., and Shipley, M. (1988). Social relationships and psychological well-being in rheumatoid arthritis. *Social Science and Medicine*, 27, 399–403.

Flor, H., Fydrich, T., and Turk, D. (1992). Efficacy of multidisciplinary pain treatment centers: A meta-analyses review. *Pain*, 49, 221–230.

Flor, H., Turk, D., and Scholz, B. (1987). Impact of chronic pain on the spouse: Marital, emotional and physical consequences. *Journal of Psychosomatic Research*, 31, 63–71.

Fordyce, W. (1995). *Back pain in the workplace*. Seattle: IASP Press.

Frank, A. (1993). Low back pain. *British Medical Journal*, 306, 901–909.

Fitzpatrick, R., Newman, S., Lamb, R., and Shipley, M. (1988). Social relationships and psychological well being in rheumatoid arthritis. *Social Science and Medicine*, 27, 399–403.

Friedman, M., McDermut, W., Solomon, D., Ryan, C., Keitner, G., and Miller, I. (1997). Family functioning and mental illness: A comparison of psychiatric and non-clinical families. *Family Process*. 36, 357–367.

Frost, H., Lamb, S., Moffett, J., Fairbank, J., and Moser, J. (1998). A fitness programme for patients with chronic low-back pain: 2 year follow-up of a randomized controlled trial. *Pain*, 75, 273–279.

Fryand, L., Wichstrom, L., Moum, T., Glennas, A., and Kvien, T. (1997). The impact of personality and social support on mental health for female patients with rheumatoid arthritis. *Social Indicators Research*, 40, 285–298.

Frymoyer, J., and Cats-Baril, W. (1991). An overview of the incidences and costs of low-back pain. *Orthopedic Clinic of North America*. 22, 263–271.

Gallagher, E. (1976). Line of extension and reconstruction in the Parsonian sociology of illness. *Social Science and Medicine*, 10, 207–218.

Gallagher, E., and Wrobel, S. (1982). The sick-role and chronic pain. In: Roy, R., and Tunks, E. (Editors). *Chronic pain: Psychosocial factors in rehabilitation*. Baltimore: Williams and Wilkins.

Gallagher, R., Rauh, L., Haugh, P., and Miltons, P. (1989). Determinants of return to work among the back pain patients. *Pain*, 39, 55–68.

Gallagher, R., Williams, R., Skelly, J., and Haugh, L. (1995). Workers' compensation and return to work in low-back pain. *Pain*, 61, 299–307.

Gatchel, R., Polatin, P., and Kinney, K. (1995). Predicting outcome of chronic back pain using clinical psychological predictors of psychopathology. *Health Psychology*, 14, 415–420.

Goldberg, R, and Wood, M. (1985). Psychotherapy for the spouses of lung cancer patients: Assessment of an intervention. *Psychotherapy and Psychosomatics*, 43: 141–150.

Goodenow, C., Reisine, S., and Grady, K. (1990). Quality of social support and associated social psychological functioning in women with rheumatoid arthritis. *Health Psychology*, 9, 266–284.

Gotlib, I., Wallace, P., and Colb, C. (1990). Marital and family therapy for depression. In: Wolman, B., and Stricker, G. (Editors). *Depressive disorders: Facts, theories and treatment methods*. New York: Wiley, pp. 396–424.

Gulhati, A., and Minty, B. (1998). Parental health attitudes, illnesses and supports and the referral of children to medical specialists. *Child Care Health and Development*. 24, 295–313.

Haley, J. (1973). *Uncommon therapy techniques of Milton Ericson*. New York: Norton

Hall, E., and Johnson, J. (1988). Depression in unemployed Swedish women. *Social Science and Medicine*. 27, 134–1355.

Hamilton, E., Hammen, C., Minasian, G., and Jones, M. (1983). Communication styles of children of mothers with affective disorders, chronic illness, medical illness and normal controls: A contextual perspective. *Journal of Abnormal Child Psychology*. 21, 51–63.

Hamilton, V., Broman, C., Hoffman, C., and Renner, D. (1990). Hard times and vulnerable people: Initial effects of plant closing on auto-workers mental health. *Journal of Health and Social Behavior*. 31,123–140.

Harvey, P. (1976). Occupational role stress within the role-set. *Free Inquiry*, 4, 77–103.

Hashemi, L., Webster, B., Clancy, E., and Volinn, E. (1997). Length of disability and cost of workers' compensation low- back claims. *Journal of Occupational and Environmental Medicine*. 39, 937–945.

Heinrich, R., and Schag, C. (1985). Stress and activity management: Group treatment for cancer patients and spouses. *Clinical and Consulting Psychology*, 53, 439–446.

Hezsen-Klemens, I., and Lapinska, E. (1984). Doctor-patient interaction, patients' health behavior and effects of treatment. *Social Science and Medicine*, 19, 9–18.

Hobdell, E. (1996). Response to "Chronic sorrow in persons with Parkinson's and their spouses." *Scholarly Inquiry for Nursing Practice*, 10, 367–370.

Holm, J., Holroyd, K., Hursey, K., and Penzien, D. (1986). The role of stress in recurrent tension headache. *Headache*, 26, 160–167.

Hudgens, J. (1979). Family oriented treatment of chronic pain. *Journal of Marital and Family Therapy*, 5, 67–78.

Inoff-Germain, G. Nottleman, E., and Radke-Yarrow, M. (1987). Relation of parental affective illness to family, dyadic, and individual functioning: An observational study of family interaction. *American Journal of Orthopsychiatry*, 67, 433–448.

Isaac, E., Minty, B., and Morrison, R. (1986). Children in care, the association with mental disorder in the parents. *British Journal of Social Work*, 16, 325–339.

Jackson, T., Iezzi, A., and Lafrenerie, K. (1998a). The impact of psychosocial features of employment status on emotional distress in chronic pain and comparison sample. *Journal of Behavioral Medicine*, 20, 241–256.

Jackson, T., Iezzi, A., Lafrenerie, K., and Harduzzi, K. (1998b). Relations of employment status to emotional distress among chronic pain patients: a pain analysis. *Clinical Journal of Pain*, 14, 55–60.

Jacob, T., and Johnson, S. (1997). Parent-child interaction among depressed fathers and mothers: Impact on child functioning. *Journal of Family Psychology*, 11, 391–409.

Jary, M. L., and Stewart, M. A. (1985). Psychiatric disorder in the parents of adopted children with aggressive conduct disorder. *Neuropsychobiology*, 13, 7–11.

Jeanneret, B., Frey, D., and Scharen, S. (1998). Chronic back pain. Schweizerische Medizinische Wochenschrift. *Journal Suisse de Medicin*, 128, 706–718.

Jensen, M., Turner, J., Romano, J., and Karoly, P. (1991). Coping with chronic pain: A critical review of the literature. *Pain*, 47, 243–249.

Johnnaon, W., Butler, R., Baldwin, M., and Burton, J., Jr. (1994). The cost effect of alternative treatments for low-back pain. AHSR & FHSK Annual Meeting Abstract Book.

Kashani, J., Burk, J., Horowitz, B., and Reid, J. (1985). Differential effect on subtype of parental major affective disorder on children. *Psychiatry Research*, 15, 195–204.

Keitner, G., Ryan, C., Miller, I., and Kohn, R. (1995). Role of the family in recovery and major depression. *American Journal of Psychiatry*, 1522, 1002–1008.

Keller, M., Beardslee, W., Dover, D., and Lovoni, P. (1986). Impact of severity and chronicity of parental affective illness on adaptive functioning and psychopathology in children. *Archives of General Psychiatry*, 43, 930–9937.

Kelly, B., Raphael, B., Judd, F., Perdices, M., Kernutt, G., Burnett, P., Dunne, M., and Burrows, G. (1998). Suicidal ideation, suicidal attempts, and HIV infection. *Psychosomatics*, 39, 405–415.

Kerns, R., and Payne, A. (1996). Treating families of chronic pain patients. In R. Gatchel and D. Turk (Editors). *Psychological approaches to pain management: Practitioners' Handbook*. New York: Guilford.

Kerns, R., and Turk, D. (1985). Depression and chronic pain: the mediating role of the spouse. *Journal of Marriage and Family*, 46, 845–852.

Klapow, J., Slater, M., Patterson, T., and Atkinson, J. (1995). Psychological factors discriminate multidimensional clinical groups of chronic low-back patients. *Pain*, 62, 349–355.

Klein, D. H., and Depue, R. A. (1985). Obsessional personality traits and risk for bipolar affective disorder: An offspring study. *Journal of Abnormal Psychology*, 94, 291–297.

Klerman, G., and Weissman, M. (1986). Interpersonal approach to understanding depression. In Millon, T., and Klerman, G. (Editors). *Contemporary directions in psychopathology*. New York: Guilford.

Klines, D., and Bolger, A. (1998). Coping with maternal depressed affect and depression: Adolescent children of depressed and well mothers. *Journal of Youth and Adolescence*, 27, 1–15.

Knight, R., Devereux, R., and Godfrey, H. (1997). Psychosocial consequences of caring for multiple sclerosis. *Journal of Clinical and Experimental Neuropsychology*, 19, 7–19.

Koch, C., Minuchen, S., and Donovan, W. (1974). A case of somatic expression of family and environmental stress. *Clinical Pediatrics*, 13, 815–818.

Koniarek, J., and Dudek, B. (1996). Social support as a buffer in the stress-burnout relationship. *International Journal of Stress Management*, 3, 99–106.

Kopp, M., Richter, R., Rainer, J., Prisca, K., Rumpold, G., and Walter, M. (1995). Differences in family functioning between patients with chronic headache and patients with chronic low-back pain. *Pain*, 63, 219–224.

Kraaimaat, F., Van Dam Baggen, C., and Bijlsma, J. (1995). Depression, anxiety and social support in rheumatoid arthritic women without and with a spouse. *Psychology and Health*, 10, 387–396.

Krentzer, J., Gerrassio, A., and Camplair, P. (1994). Patient correlates of caregivers' distress and family functioning after traumatic brain injury. *Brain Injury*, 8, 211–230.

Kriegsman, D., Penninx, B., and van Eijk, J. (1994). Chronic disease in the elderly and its impact on the family: A review of the literature. *Arthritis Care and Research, Family Systems Medicine*, 12, 249–267.

Kriegsman, D., van Eijk, J., Penninx, B., and Deeg, D. (1997). Does family support buffer the impact of specific chronic diseases on mobility in community dwelling elderly? *Disability and Rehabilitation: An International Multi-disciplinary Journal*, 19, 71–83.

Kunzer, M. (1986). Structural family therapy with chronic pain patients. *Issues in Medical Health Nursing*, 8, 213–222.

LaMata, R., Gingras, G., and Wittkower, E. (1960). Impact of sudden, severe disablement of the father upon the family. *Canadian Medical Association Journal*, 82, 1015–1020.

Lambert, V., Lambert, C., Kipple, G., and Mewshaw, E. (1989). Social support, hardiness and psychological well-being in women with arthritis. *Image: Journal of Nursing Scholarship*, 21, 128–131.

Latha, K., Bhat, S., and D'Souza, P. (1994). Attempted suicide and recent stressful events: A report from India. *CRISIS*, 15, 136.

Leavitt, F., and Sweet, B. (1986). Characteristics and frequency of malingering among patients with low back pain. *Pain*, 25, 357–364.

LeFort, S., Gray-Donald, M., Rowet, K., and Jeans, M-E. (1998). Randomized controlled trial of a community based psycho education program for the self-management of chronic pain. *Pain*, 74, 297–306.

Lewy, E. (1940). Contribution to the problem of compensation neuroses. *Bulletin of the Menninger Clinic*, 4, 88–92.

Liebman, R., Honig, P., and Berger, M. (1976). An integrated treatment for pain. *Family Process*, 15, 397–405.

Lieberman, M., and Fisher, L. (1995). The impact of chronic illness on the health and well-being of family members. *Gerontologist*, 35, 94–105.

Lieff, J. (1982). Eight reasons why doctors fear the elderly, chronic illness, and death. *Journal of Transpersonal Psychology*, 14, 47–60.

Lindgren, C. (1996). Chronic sorrow in persons with Parkinson's and their spouses. *Scholarly Inquiry for Nursing Practice*, 10, 351–366.

Linn, R., Allen, K., and Willer, B. (1994). Affective symptoms in the chronic stage of traumatic brain injury. *Brain Injury*, 8, 135–147.

Linn, M., Sanfer, R., and Stein, S. (1985). Effects of unemployment on mental and physical health. *American Journal of Public Health*, 75, 502–506.

Linton. S. (1990). The socioeconomic impact of chronic back pain: Is anyone helping? *Pain*. 75, 163–168.

Linton, S. (1998). Risk-factors for neck and back pain in a working population in Sweden. *Work and Stress*, 4, 41–49.

Lyster, G., and Youssef, H. (1995). Attempted suicide in a catchment area of Ireland: A comparison of an urban and rural population. *European Journal of Psychiatry*, 9, 22–27.

Liu, A., and Byrne. E. (1995). Cost of care for ambulatory patients with low-back pain. *Journal of Family Practice*, 40, 449–455.

Luchetta, T. (1995). Parental work role salience, every day problems and distress: A prospective analyses of specific vulnerability among multiple role women. *Women and Health*, 22, 21–50.

Madanes, C. (1981). Strategic family therapy. San Francisco: Jossey-Bass.

Manne, S., and Zaruta, A. (1989). Spouse criticism and support: Their association with coping and psychological adjustment among women with rheumatoid arthritis. *Journal of Personality and Social Psychology*, 56, 608–617.

Marcoux, R. (1994). Invisible workers do not strike: A reflection on child labor in the urban milieu of Mali. *Labor, Capital and Society*, 27, 296–319.

Martin, P., and Nathan, P. (1987). Differential prevalence rates for headaches: A function of stress and social support. *Headache*, 27, 392–333.

Martin, P., and Soon, K. (1993). The relationship between perceived stress, social support, and chronic headache. *Headache*, 33, 307–314.

Martin, P., and Theunissen, C. (1993). The role of life-event stress, coping and social support in chronic headache. *Headache*, 33, 301–306.

McFarlane, A., Norman, G., Streiner, D., and Roy, R. (1983). The process of social stress: stable, reciprocal and mediating relationships. *Journal of Health and Social Behavior*, 24, 160–173.

McIntosh, G., Melles, T., and Hall, H. (1995). Guidelines for the identification of barriers to rehabilitation of back injuries. *Journal of Occupational Rehabilitation*, 5, 195–201.

McKenna, S., and Payne, R. (1989). Comparison of the general health questionnaire and the Nottingham Health Profile on a study of unemployed and re-employed men. Family Practice, 6, 3–8.

Mendelson, G. (1984). Compensation pain complaints and psychological disturbance. *Pain*, 5, 173–178.

Melamed, B., and Brenner, G. (1990). Social support and chronic medical stress: An interaction-based approach. *Journal of Social and Clinical Psychology*, 9, 104–117.

Melzack, R., Katz, J., and Jeans, M. (1985). The role of compensation on chronic pain. *Pain*, 23, 101–112.

Merskey, H., and Magni, G. (1990). Psychological techniques in the treatment of chronic pain. In Miller, T. (Editor). *Chronic Pain*. Madison, CT: International University Press.

Mikail, S., and von Bayer, C. (1990). Pain, somatic focus and emotional adjustment in children of chronic headache sufferers and controls. *Social Science and Medical*, 31, 51–59.

Miller, E., Berrios, G., and Politynska, B. (1996). Caring for someone with Parkinson's disease. *International Journal of Geriatric Psychiatry*, 11, 263–268.

Miller, I., Epstein, N., Bishop, D., and Keitner, G. (1985). The McMaster family assessment device: Reliability and validity. *Journal of Marital and Family Therapy*, 11, 345–356.

Miller, I., Keitner, G., Whisman, M., and Ryan, C. (1992). Depressed patients with dysfunctional families: Description and course of illness. *Journal of Abnormal Psychology*, 101, 637–646.

Mitchelmore, M. (1996). The psychosocial implications of back injury at work. *Nursing Standard*, 10, 33–38.

Mohamed, S., Weisz, G., Cope, N., and Jones, J. (1978). The relationship of chronic pain to depression, marital and family dynamics. *Pain*, 5, 282–292.

Morrell, S., Taylor, R., Quine, S., and Kerr, C. (1993). Suicide and unemployment in Australia. *Social Science and Medicine*, 36, 749–756.

Morris, P., Robinson, R., Raphael, B., and Bishop, D. (1991). The relationship between the perception of social support and post-stroke depression in hospitalized patients. *Psychiatry*, 54, 306–316.

Naidoo, P., and Pillay, Y. (1994). Correlations among general stress, family environment, psychological distress, and pain experience. *Perceptual and Motor Skills*, 78, 1291–1296.

Nicassio, P., and Radojevic, V. (1993). Models of family functioning and their contribution to patients outcomes in chronic pain. *Motivation and Emotion*, 17, 295–316.

Nicassio, P., Radojevic, V., Schofield-Smith, K., and Dwyer, K. (1995). The contribution of family cohesion and pain coping process to depressive symptoms in fibromyalgia. *Annals of Behavioral Medicine*, 17, 349–356.

O'Brien, R., Wineman, N., and Nealon, N. (1995). Correlates of the caregiving process in multiple sclerosis. *Scholarly Inquiry for Nursing Practice*, 9, 323–338.

Okifuji, A., Turk, D., and Kaloukalani, D. (1998). Clinical outcome and economic evaluation of multidisciplinary pain clinic. In: Block, A., Kremer, E., and Fernandez, E. (Editors). *Handbook of pain syndrome: Biopsychosocial perspectives*. Mawhaw: NJ, Lawrence Erlbaum Associates.

Parker, J., and Wright, G. (1997). Assessment and quality of life in rheumatic diseases. *Arthritis Care and Research*, 10, 406–412.

Parsons, T. (1951). *The social system*. Glencoe, Illinois: Free Press.

Payne, B., and Norfleet, M. (1986). Chronic pain and the family: A review. *Pain*, 26, 1–22.

Penninx, B., Kriegsman, D., van Eijk, J., Boeke, J., and Deeg, D. (1996). Differential effect of social support on the course of chronic disease: A criteria-based literature study. *Families, Systems and Health*, 14, 223–244.

Penninx, B., Van Tilburg, T., Deeg, D., and Kriegsman, D. (1997). Direct and buffer effects of social support and personal coping resources in individuals with arthritis. *Social Science and Medicine*, 44, 393–402.

Peterson, K. (1985). Psychological adjustment of the family caregivers: Home hemodialysis as an example. *Social Work in Health Care*, 10, 15–32.

Petrie, K., and Brook, R. (1992). Sense of cohesiveness, self-esteem, depression and hopelessness as correlates of reattempting suicide. *British Journal of Clinical Psychiatry*, 31, 293–300.

Pfingston, M., Hilderbrandt, J., Liebing, E., Franz, C., and Saur, P. (1997). Effectiveness of multi-modal treatment for chronic low-back pain. *Pain*, 73, 77–85.

Plant, H., Richardson, J., Stubbs, J., Lynch, L., Elwood, D., Slevin, M., and DeHass, H. (1987). Evaluation of support groups for cancer patients and families. *British Journal of Hospital Medicine*, 38, 317–322.

Potts, M., Mazzuca, S., and Brandt, K. (1986). Views of patients and physicians regarding the importance of various aspects of arthritis treatment: Correlation with healthy status and patient satisfaction. *Patient Education and Counseling*, 8, 125–134.

Prince, S., and Jacobson, N. (1995). Couple and family therapy for depression. In: Beckham, E., and Leber, W. (Editors). *Handbook of depression*. New York: Guilford Press.

Raphael, K., Dohrenwend, B., and Marbach, J. (1990). Illness and injury among children of temporomandibular pain and dysfunction syndrome. *Pain*, 40, 61–64.

Reisine, S., and Fifled, J. (1995). Family work demands, employment demands and depressive symptoms in women with rheumatoid arthritis. *Women and Health*, 22, 22–45.

Retzer, A., Simon, F., Weber, G., and Stricklin, H. (1991). A follow-up study of manic-depressive and schzioaffective psychosis after systemic family therapy. *Family Process*, 30, 139–153.

Revenson, T., and Majerovitz, S. (1991). The effects of chronic illness on the spouse: Social resources as stress buffers. *Arthritis Care and Research*, 4, 63–72.

Rickard, K. (1988). The occurrence of maladaptive health behaviors and teach rated conduct problems in children of chronic low-back patients. *Journal of Behavioral Medicine*, 11, 107–116.

Ricke, S., Chara, P., and Johnson, M. (1995). Work-hardening: Evidence for success of a program. *Psychological Reports*, 77, 1077–1078.

Rife, J., and First, R. (1989). Discouraged older workers: an exploration study. *International Journal of Aging and Human Development*, 29, 195–203.

Roberts, B., Matecjyck, M., and Anthony, M. (1996). The effects of social support on the relationship of functional limitations and pain to depression. *Arthritis Care and Research*, 9, 67–73.

Rodrigue, J., and Hoffman, R. (1994). Caregivers of adults with cancer: Multidimensional correlates of psychological distress. *Journal of Clinical Psychology in Medical Settings*, 1, 231–244.

Romano, J., Turner, J., and Jensen, M. (1997). The family environment in chronic pain patients: Comparison to controls and relationship to patient functioning. *Journal of Clinical Psychology in Health Settings*, 4, 383–395.

Rowat, K., and Knafl, K. (1985). Living with chronic pain: The spouses' perspective. *Pain*, 23, 259–271.

Roy, R. (1988). Impact of chronic pain on marital partners. In: Dubner, R., Gebhart, T., and Bond, M. (Editors). *Pain research and clinical management*. Amsterdam: Elsevier, pp. 286–297.

Roy, R. (1989). *Chronic pain and the family: A problem-centered perspective*. New York: Human Sciences Press.

Roy, R. (1990). Physical illness, chronic pain and family therapy. In: Tunks, E., Bellissimmo, A., and Roy, R. (Editors), *Chronic pain: Psychosocial factors in rehabilitation*. 2nd ed. Melbourne, FL: Krieger.

Roy, R. (1990). Chronic pain and "effective" family functioning: A re-examination of the McMaster Model of Family Functioning. *Contemporary Family Therapy*, 12, 489–503.

Roy, R. (1990-91). Impact of parental illness on children. *Social Science and Social Work Review*, 2, 109–121.

Roy, R., and Frankel, H. (1995). How good is family therapy: A reassessment. Toronto: University of Toronto Press.

Roy, R., and Thomas, M. (1989). Nature of marital relations among chronic pain patients. *Contemporary Family Therapy*, 11, 277–284.

Roy, R., Thomas, M., Mogilevsky, I., and Cook, A. (1994). Influence of parental chronic pain on children: Preliminary observations. *Headache Quarterly*, 5, 20–26.

Rudas. N., Tondo, L., Musio, A., and Spada, S. (1991). Depressive features in unemployed individuals. *Minerva Psychiatry*. 32, 229–232.

Rueveni, U. (1990). Empowering chronic headache sufferers. *Contemporary Family Therapy*, 12, 505–514.

Rutter, M. (1966). *Children of sick parents: An environmental and psychiatric study*. London: Oxford University Press.

Rutter, M. (1989). Pathways from childhood to adult life. *Journal of Clinical Psychology and Psychiatry*, 30, 23–51.

Saaijaervi, S. (1990). Effectiveness of psychotherapy in low-back pain. *Psychiatrica Fennica*, 23, 95–102.

Saarijaervi, S., Hyyppae, M., Lehtinen, V., and Alanen, E. (1990). Chronic low-back pain patient and spouse. *Journal of Psychosomatic Research*, 34, 117–122.

Sanders, S., and Brena, S. (1993). Empirically derived chronic pain patient sub-groups: The utility of multi-dimensional clustering to identify differential treatment effects. *Pain*, 54, 51–56.

Schanberg, L., Keefe, F., Lefevre, J., Kredich, D., and Gil, K. (1998). Social context of pain in children with juvenile primary fibromyalgia syndrome: Parental pain history and family environment. *Clinical Journal of Pain*, 14, 107–115.

Scharloo, M., Kaptein, A., Weinman, J., Hazes, J., Williems, L., Bergman, W., and Rooilmans, H. (1998). Illness perceptions, coping, and functioning in patients with rheumatoid arthritis, chronic obstructive pulmonary disease and psoriasis. *Journal of Psychosomatic Research*, 44, 573–585.

Schiaffino, K., and Revenson, T. (1995). Relative contribution of spousal support and illness appraisals to depressed mood in arthritis patients. *Arthritis Care and Research*, 8, 80–87.

Schulman, J. (1988). Using a coping approach in the management of children with conversion reactions. *Journal of American Academy of Child and Adolescent Psychiatry*, 27, 785–788.

Schulz, R., Newsom, J., Mittleman, M., Burton, L., Hirsch, C., and Jackson, S. (1997). Health effects of caregiving: An ancillary study of the Cardiovascular Health Study. *Annals of Behavioral Medicine*, 19, 110–116.

Schwartz, L. (1946). Neuroses following head and brain injury. *Harper Hospital Bulletin*, 4, 179–183.

Schwartz, L., Slater, M., Birchler, G., and Atkinson, J. (1991). Depression in spouses of chronic pain patients and the role of the patients' pain, anger and marital satisfaction. *Pain*, 44, 61–67.

Shanfield, S., Herman, E., Cope, N., and Jones, J. (1979). Pain and the marital relationship: *PsychiatricDistress*, 7, 343–351.

Shaw, W., Semple, S., Ho, S., Irwin, M., Hanger, R., Grant, I., and Patterson, T. (1997). Longitudinal analyses of multiple indicators of health decline among spousal caregivers. *Annals of Behavioral Medicine*, 19, 101–109.

Sherbourne, C., and Hays, R. (1990). Marital status, social support, and health transitions in chronic disease patients. *Journal of Health and Social Behavior*, 31, 328–343.

Simmonds, M., Kumar, S., and Cechelt, E. (1996). Psychological factors in disabling low-back pain: Cause or consequence? *Disability and Rehabilitation*, 18, 161–168.

Simmonds, M., and Sharwan, K. (1996). Does knowledge of patient's workers' compensation status influence clinical judgement? *Journal of Occupational Rehabilitation*, 6, 93–107.

Simonsick, E. (1993). Relationship between husband's health status and the mental health of older women. *Journal of Aging and Health*, 5, 319–337.

Smith, R. (1985). "I really feel ashamed": How does unemployment lead to poorer mental health? *Psychological Medicine*, 15, 789–793.

Smith, R. (1998). Impact of migraine on the family. *Headache*, 38, 423–426.

Soederman, E., and Lisspers, J. (1997). Diagnosing depression with physical diseases using the Beck Depression Inventory. *Scandinavian Journal of Behavior Therapy*, 26, 102–112.

Stang, P., Von Korff, M., and Galer, B. (1998). Reduced labor force participation among primary care patients with headache. *Journal of General Internal Medicine*, 13, 296–302.

Steele, R., Tripp, G., Kotchick, B., Summers, P., and Forehand, R. (1997). Family member's uncertainness about parental chronic illness: The relationship of neurophilia and HIV infection to child functioning. *Journal of Pediatric Psychology*, 22, 577–591.

Stevenson, G. (1932). On being a patient. *Mental Hygiene*, 16, 37–55.

Stoleru, S., Nottlemann, E., Belmont, B., and Ronsaville, D. (1997). Sleep problem in children of affectively ill mothers. *Journal of Child Psychology and Psychiatry and Allied Disciplines*, 38, 831–8841.

Stratton, K., Maisick, R., Wrigley, J., White, M., Johnson, P., and Fine, P. (1996). Barriers to return to work among persons unemployed due to arthritis and musculoskeletal disorders. *Arthritis and Rheumatism*, 39, 101–109.

Subramanian, K. (1991). The multidimensional impact of chronic pain on the spouse: A pilot study. *Social Work in Health Care*, 15, 47–61.

Tait, R., Chibnall, J., and Richardson, W. (1990). Litigation and employment status: Effects on patients with chronic pain. *Pain*, 43, 37–46.

Tan, V., Cheatle, M., Mackin, S., Moburg, P., and Esterhai, J. (1997). Goal setting as a predictor of return to work in a population of chronic musculoskeletal chronic pain patients. *International Journal of Neuroscience*, 92, 161–170.

Tarullo, L., DeMulder, E., Martinez, P., and Radke-Yarrow, K. (1994). Dialogues with pre-adolescents and adolescents: Mother-child interaction patterns in affectively ill and well dyads. *Journal of Abnormal Psychology*, 22, 33–51.

Teasell, R., and Finestone, H. (1999). Socio-economic factors and work disability: Clues to managing chronic pain diseases. *Pain Research and Management*, 4, 89–92.

Teti, D., Gelfand, D., Messinger, D., and Isabella, R. (1995). Maternal depression and the quality of early attachment: An examination of infants, pre-schoolers and their mothers. *Developmental Psychology*, 31, 364–376.

Theorell, T., Haggmark, C., and Eneroth, P. (1987). Psycho-endocrinological reaction in female relatives of cancer patients. *Acta Oncologia (Sweden)*, 26, 419–424.

Thomas, M., and Roy, R. (1999). *The changing nature of pain complaints over lifetime*. New York: Plenum.

Thomas, S. (1977). Distressing aspects of women's roles, vicarious stress and health consequences. *Mental Health Nursing*, 18, 539–557.

Thompson, S., Bundek, N., and Shobolew-Shubin, A. (1990). The caregivers of stroke patients. *Journal of Applied Social Psychology*, 20, 115–129.

Thompson, S., Medvene, L., and Freedman, D. (1995). Caregiving in the close relationships of cardiac patients: Exchange power and attributional perspectives on caregiver resentment. *Personal Relationship*, 2, 125–142.

Thompson, S., Shobolew-Shubin, A., Graham, M., and Janigian, A. (1989). Psychological adjustment following stroke. *Social Science and Medicine*, 28, 239–247.

Tisher, M., Tonge, B., and Horne, D. (1994). Childhood depression and parental depression. *Australian and New Zealand Journal of Psychiatry*, 28, 635–641.

Tollison, D. (1991). Comprehensive treatment approach for lower back pain workers' compensation injuries. *Journal of Occupational Rehabilitation*, 1, 281–287.

Trief, P., Carnrike, C., and Drudge, O. (1995). Chronic pain and depression: Is social support relevant? *Psychological Reports*, 76, 227–236.

Tunks, E. (1990). Chronic pain and the occupational role, Part 1. In: Tunks, E., Bellissimo, A., and Roy, R. (Editors). *Chronic pain: Psychosocial factors in rehabilitation*. 2nd revised ed. Melbourne, FL: Krieger.

Twemlow, S., Bradshaw, S., Coyne, L., and Lerma, B. (1997). Patterns of utilization of medical care and perceptions between doctor and patient with chronic illness including chronic fatigue syndrome. *Psychological Reports*, 80, 643–658.

Valat, J., Goupille, P., and Vedene, V. (1997). Low-back pain: Risk factors for chronicity. *Review Rheumatology*, English Edition, 64, 189–1994.

Van Tudler, M., Koes, R., and Bouter, L. (1995). Cost of illness study of back pain in the Netherlands. *Pain*, 62, 233–240.

Vaughn, C., and Leff, J. (1976). The influence of family and social factors on the course of psychiatric illness: A comparison of schizophrenic and depressed neurotic patients. *British Journal of Psychiatry*, 159, 383–389.

Viinamaeki, H., Koskela, K., Niskanen, L., and Arnkill, R. (1993). Unemployment, financial stress and mental well-being. A factory closure study. *European Journal of Psychiatry*, 7, 95–102.

Vinokur, A., Price, R., and Caplan, R. (1996). Hard times and hurtful partner: How financial strain affects depression and relationship satisfaction of unemployed persons and their spouses. *Journal of Personality and Social Psychology*, 71, 166–179.

Violon, A. (1982). Becoming a chronic pain patient. In: Roy, R., and Tunks, E. (Editors). *Chronic pain: Psychosocial factors in rehabilitation*. Baltimore: Williams & Wilkins.

Vitaliano, P., Dougherty, C., and Siegler, C. (1994). Biopsychosocial risks for cardiovascular disease in spouses caregivers of persons with Alzheimer's disease. In: Abeles, R., and Gift, H. (Editors). *Aging and quality of life*. New York: Springer.

Volinn, E. (1986). Sociological factors and chronic pain. Paper presented at a meeting of the Society for the Study of Social Problems.

Volinn, E., Turezyn, K., and Loser, J. (1991). Theories of back-pain and health care utilization. *Neurosurgery Clinics of North America*, 2, 739–748.

Von Korff, M., Ormel, J., Keefe, F., and Dworkin, S. (1992). Grading the severity of chronic pain. *Pain*, 50, 133–149.

Waddell, G. (1996). Low back pain: a twentieth century health care enigma. *Spine*, 21, 280–2825.

Walhagen, M., and Brod, M. (1997). Perceived control and well-being in Parkinson's disease. *Western Journal of Nursing Research*, 19, 11–31.

Waltz, M., Kriegel, W., and van Pad Bosch, P. (1998). The social environment and health in rheumatoid arthritis: Marital quality predicts individual variability in pain severity. *Arthritis Care and Research*, 11, 356–374.

Waring, E., Chamberlain, C., Carver, C., and Stalker, C. (1995). A pilot study of marital therapy as treatment for depression. *American Journal of Psychiatry*, 23, 3–10.

Watson, W., Bell, J., and Wright, L. (1992). Osteophytes and marital fights. *Family Systems Medicine*, 10, 423–435.

Webster, B., and Snook, S. (1990). The cost of compensable low back pain. *Journal of Occupational Medicine*, 32, 13–15.

Weinberg, M., and Tronick, E. (1998). The impact of maternal psychiatric illness on infant development. *Journal of Clinical Psychiatry*, 59 (Suppl.2), 53–61.

Weinberger, M., Tierney, W., Boober, P., and Hiner, S. (1990). Social support, stress and functional status in patients with osteoarthritis. *Social Science and Medicine*, 30, 503–508.

Weissman, M., Warner, V., Wickramaratne, P., Moreau, D., and Olfson, M. (1987). Offspring of depressed parents: 10 years later. *Archives of General Psychiatry*, 54, 932–940.

Welz, W. (1968–69). Traumatic neuroses and compensation neuroses. *Pennsylvania Psychiatric Quarterly*, 8, 3–15.

Wesley, W., and Epstein, N. (1970). *The silent majority*. San Francisco: Jossey-Bass.

Williams, A. (1998). A group for the adult daughters of mentally ill mothers: Looking backwards and forwards. *British Journal of Medical Psychology*, 7, 73–83.

Worsham, N., Compass, B., and Ey, S. (1997). Children's coping with parental illness. In: Wollchin, S., and Sandler, R. (Editors). *Handbook of children's coping: Linking theory and intervention*. New York: Plenum.

Ystgaard, M., Tambs, K., and Dalgard, O. (1999). Life stress, social support and psychological distress in late adolescence: A longitudinal study. *Social Psychiatry and Psychiatric Epidemiology*, 34, 12–19.

INDEX